Shannon Fernandes

PRECISION ATTACHMENTS

Attachments in dentistry

LAP LAMBERT Academic Publishing

Publisher:
LAP LAMBERT Academic Publishing
is a trademark of
International Book Market Service Ltd., member of OmniScriptum Publishing Group
17 Meldrum Street, Beau Bassin 71504, Mauritius

ISBN: 978-620-0-52900-8

INTRODUCTION

"By definition, the term precision denotes the quality or state of being precise".

Maintenance of periodontal health is one of the essentials when striving for a favorable prognosis in prosthetic dentistry. The achievement of such a state, however, often turns out to be difficult.[1] Misconceptions about the use of intracoronally retained prosthesis have discouraged many practitioners to use them in their dental practices. However the prosthodontist who employs this form of treatment quickly learns its benefits in providing patients with an esthetic prosthesis.

Precision attachments are at times said to be a connecting link between the fixed and removable type of partial dentures because it incorporates features common to both types of construction. Precision attachments in dentistry is a means of bodily function for a removable bridge or partial dentures (Steiger and Boitel).

Precision attachments retain and attach a removable bridge or partial denture on natural teeth vital or nonvital.

Some serve as retainers for full overdentures where few abutments remain. The main purpose of precision attachment besides its retention is its cover up within or under a restoration as an esthetically better option to a visible metal clasp retainer.

Development of precision attachments are two basic objectives. These are :

1. To provide the desired platform for the available tooth support.

2. To distribute the load to the teeth as far as possible to by the appliance.

In order to achieve these two objectives precision attachments have been constructed into two halves, a matrix and a patrix. The two halves being arranged in a way that they articulate with one another to form a very precise but a separable joint.[4] The two parts are also referred to as the male and female parts. The abutment retainers houses a slot (female) which fits the male part into it. Its synonyms are Internal attachments, frictional attachments, slotted attachments, parallel attachments, and key and keyway attachments.

An attachment is a precision connector made up of two or more parts. One part is connected to a tooth, root or implant. The other is connected to an artificial prosthesis to provide mechanical connection between the two (Michael Sheering Lucas and Paul Martin). An attachment is a mechanical device for the fixation, retention and stabilization of a dental prosthesis.[7] Precision attachment may be prefabricated by a manufacturer or in the dental laboratory. The manufactured type is made of precious metal. The fit of the two working elements is machined to very close tolerance and is more precise in construction than the laboratory type. The patrix takes the shape of a "T" or "H" which fits an appropriately shaped slot (matrix). The female attachment is fitted into the restoration within the contour of tooth either by casting the gold to it or placing it in a prepared receptacle in the restoration and by attaching the two together with solder.[2] The male and female parts are matched to interlock together and provide direct retention for the partial denture.[1]

The semiprecision attachment is referred to as „precision rest" „milled rest" or „internal rest". This type of retainer takes the form of a dovetail shaped keyway built into the proximal surfaces of wax pattern of a gold crown.6

DEFINITIONS

Precision attachment

1. A retainer consisting of a metal receptacle (matrix) and a closely fitting part (patrix). The matrix is usually contained within the normal or expanded contours of the crown on the abutment tooth and the patrix is attached to a pontic or the removable partial denture frame work (Glossary of prosthodontic terms Sixth Edition 1994).

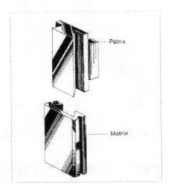

Synonyms

Internal attachment, parallel attachment, frictional attachment, key and key way attachment, slotted attachment.

2. A retainer used in fixed and removable partial denture construction consisting of a metal receptacle and a closely fitting part, the former is usually contained within the normal or expanded contours of the crown of the abutment tooth, and the latter is attached to a pontic or to the denture frame work.[6]

3. Implies a partly or wholly machined device consisting of a male and female components which is used in restorative dentistry to retain removable or semi-removable prosthesis.[1]

4. Are wholly or partially machined accessories used in dentistry for the retention of removable or semi-removable prosthesis (G.E.Ray precision attachments).

INTRACORONAL PRECISION ATTACHMENTS

The bulk of the soldered or cast on portion of the joint lies within the contours of the treated teeth (G.E. Ray – Precision Attachments).

EXTRACORONAL PRECISION ATTACHMENTS

Are used to join a prosthesis to a retainer, part of all of their mechanisms is outside the anatomical contour of the retainer.63

Winder and Parr invented devices which are attachments both in principle and design, credit is usually given to George Evans 1888 for introduction of precision attachment retainer system.

Early pioneers such as Peeso (1894), Carr (1898) Goslee (1913) Gilmore (1913), Fossume (1906), Bennett (1904), Brown, Bryant, Conduit, Golobin, Kelley, McCollum, Morgan, Roach, Sorensen, Supplee (all from Unites States of America) were highly innovative with their deigns, had only limited insight into the biologic dynamics of fixed and removable prosthodontics as related to the periodontal apparatus.

Development of intracoronal and extracoronal attachments has been traced from antiquity to modern times. The history of intracornal retainer systems began in ancient times with the Phoenicians, between the 4th and 5th century B.C. where artisans and Goldsmiths created artificial replacements. Usually anterior teeth were replaced with extracted human teeth and these were attached with gold wire to each other and to the adjacent remaining teeth. During the old kingdom

(3100.2181 BC) in Egypt anterior replacements were created by artisans who threaded gold wire through extracted teeth and then wrapped the gold wire around these replacements and anchored them to the adjacent remaining teeth. About the 4th century BC, the Etruscans constructed fixed removable prostheses replacing one or more missing teeth by using soft, pure gold bands that were soldered together, surrounding the remaining teeth and carrying the replacement.

Dubois De Chemant anchored the partial dentures with clasps in its simplest form and developed it later. Delabarre had constructed a kind of supported prosthesis in 1820. a saddle shaped spring was introduced by the London dentist. De la Fons 1826 which exerted its force partially in the open position and partially in the closed and extended within the row of teeth between the points of contact similar to the Jacksons clasp.

The Griswold attachment introduced in 1889 was a triangular tube and sleeve. The inner patrix was soldered to the abutment restoration and the outer matrix was attached to the gold or vulcanite denture base.

Bryant in 1894 fabricated an attachment system by soldering iridoplatinum wire guide posts, the size of a large pin to the proximal surfaces of the abutment crowns.

The conduit attachments 1895 was a circular type of system. It consisted of a tubular patrix open at the side facing the edentuolous area and at its ends. The patrix was soldered to the abutment restoration.

Morgans attachment was patented in 1901. it consisted of a "keeper", the matrix which was soldered to the abutment restoration as an extracoronal device.

Roach in 1904 published an article describing as hand made intracoronal attachment system. Chayes in 1908 stated that the biological principle that govern function of normal teeth could not be violated without consequences. He stressed the importance of movement of teeth in their resilient socket during function.

Ash 1912 introduced the split bar attachment system. This retentive system was laboratory fabricated and required that the abutment teeth be nonvital. The Yiridian intracoronal attachment system introduced in 1918 consisted of split post and split bar device. J. Wright Beach in 1916 published the rationale for incorporating a lug rest in al removable partial dentures. He argued that the lug rest was an integral part of the clasp to maintain the retainer in its pre-determined position.

Henry W. Gillett developed a deep rest system for use with movable removable partial dentures in 1923. This was the first semiprecision attachment. It was laboratory fabricated and had a solid metal deep rest that fit into a rest seat carved into the abutment restoration.

Victor H. Jackson in New York used only round spring action, plantinum, iridum wire for his treatment aid designated as "crib". In 1887 he developed in into a universal tool. The appliance was fastened with clasps which overlapped the interdental space between crowns of premolar and molar.

Without doubt, the most important character in the development of precision attachment dentistry was Dr. Herman. E. S. Chayes He can be called the father of precision intra coronal retainer. Chayes was born in 1880 in Poland, from where he emigrated to New York in 1893. before entering dental college, he worked in a corset factory where the invented a detectable suspender device which formed the fundamental feature of his dental attachment. Chayes qualified with honours at New York college of dentistry in 1900. between 1908 and 1910, he invented a parallelometer and in 1912 he deigned Chayes attachment. This was the first attachment to be placed in the general market and still forms the basic pattern for most of the modern attachments. It is an intracoronal mesiodistal attachment.

Since then, the technology of attachments have progressed at such a rapid rate, that from a very T shaped attachments and bar attachments (1915-1935) various attachments of most diversified designs are available today.

In Europe, particularly Switzerland known as the country of watch makers and fine mechanics development in the field of attachment picked momentum before, during and after the second would war.

Steiger, Boitel, Muller and Biaggi were the force runners.

In 1959, Alfred Steiger and Raoul B. Boitel perfected channel shoulder – pin (C.S.P. system)

In Europe, laboratory made attachments because known during first world war, when readymade attachments from United States were unobtainable.

GOALS

The goals for fabrication of precision attachment prosthesis are as follows :

a. To be replaceable and removable without stress or stain on the abutment teeth.

b. To allow for normal anatomic contour to the abutment teeth.

c. To provide many years of comfort to the patient.

d. To be made of materials, compatible with oral tissues.

e. To be resistant to abrasion

f. To be resistant to corrosion

g. To be esthetically acceptable by patients

h. To require minimal amount of tooth structure removal

i. To be hygienically clean

INDICATIONS AND CONTRA INDICATIONS

Indications

1. Movable joints in fixed movable bridge work

2. As stress breaker in free end saddles and in bridges

3. Intracoronal attachments are effective retainers for re-movable partial dentures

4. As a connector for sectional dentures

5. Sections of a fixed prosthesis may be connected with intracoronal attachments

6. To lock a connector joining a saddle on the opposite side of the arch

7. Periodontal involvement that contraindicates fixed partial dentures

8. Labial clasp arms which would be displayed in the ante-rior part of the mouth and would be esthetically unpleas-ing

Contraindications

1. Sick and the senile (prosthesis with attachments must be inserted along one precise path of insertion, the pa-tient must posses an average degree of manual skill).

2. Periodontosis

3. High caries rate

4. Inadequate space to accommodate the attachments (in teeth that are very narrow facio-lingually).

ADVANTAGES AND DISADVANTAGES

Advantages

1. The labial or buccal clasp arm can be eliminated altogether making it esthetic excellent for the denture especially in the maxillary arch.

2. Precision attachments are less traumatic to the abutment teeth than conventional clasps. Precision attachment is located deep within the confines of the tooth therefore all stress is directed along long axis of the teeth.

Disadvantages

1. The tooth may have to be extensively cut to provide space to accommodate intracoronal attachment

2. A bulge is created in the crown by intra coronal attachment

3. The attachment is subject to wear as a result of friction between metal parts. As wear occurs, male portion fits

more loosely thus permitting excessive movement and threat of injury to abutment teeth.

4. The extra coronal type of retainer extends out from the tooth near the gingival border which can cause a gingival irritation followed by inflammation.

5. The extracoronal type of attachment must occupy the space immediately adjacent to abutment tooth, which is precisely where a replacement tooth should ideally be positioned.

PRECISION VERSUS SEMIPRECISION

Advantages of precision attachments

1. Standardization of sizing within an individual manufacturer"s line providing easy inter changeability of male and female attachments for replacement or repair purposes.

2. Lesser degree of technical competency

3. Pre fabricated precision attachment has the advantage of being fabricated from metal alloys which are harder and more wear resistant.

Disadvantages

1. Expensive and not economical for the patient

2. Poor proximal contour occurring on restoration

3. Proximal, parallel sides striker plate impinges on the gingiva when an attempt is made to achieve maximum possible attachment.

Advantages of semi precision attachments

1. Greater adaptability to a variety of clinical situations

2. Variation in tooth size and shape are easily accommodated

3. More economical

4. Crown contour is better achieved in the gingival area with laboratory fabricated precision attachment

Disadvantages of semi precision attachments

1. Greater degree of skill is required

2. Repair and replacement is more difficult than with prefabricated precision attachment because of the lack of interchangeability of custom attachment.

3. The long-term wear of custom made attachments becomes a problem because of the softness of the gold alloys used.

Intracoronal attachments

These type of attachements are within the anatomical contour of the crown of natural tooth. They provide rigid connection between the saddle and abutment tooth and provides frictional contact between the parallel surfaces of the flange and slot. Modern attachments utilize a H-shaped flange which is stronger and has double the frictional surfaces areas of the earlier T-shaped flange. At least three to four of these attachments are included in denture and they have to be aligned so that all the slots are parallel to each other to ensure precise insertion and removal.

The main problem faceed in the use of intra coronal attachments is providing sufficient space within the contour of the abutment tooth to accommodate the female part. It is essential that this part does not project over the gingival margin nor interfere with the occlusal contacts. Hence, adequate depth of preparation is required anterior-posteriorly to avoid the gingival impingement and sufficient height must be available to provide as large an area of frictional contact as possible between the slot and flange.[8]

Intracoronal attachments are indicated for bounded saddles unilateral dentures in class III when tooth contours are unsuitable for clasps. When these are used for free and saddle dentures, the rigid connection between the denture and the abutment teeth requires that at least two teeth are splinted together on either side to form double abutments and if only six anterior teeth remain they should all be splinted together to form one abutment.

To reduce the load on the attachments it is advantageous to incorporate into the denture a rigid lingual bracing arm to the most distal abutment tooth. This arm will provide more stability to the denture and will also provide a guiding plane for the path of insertion.

Extra coronal attachment

These attachments have all or a part of their mechanism lying outside the contour of the crown of the abutment tooth. As a result loads falling on the tooth via the attachment are applied outside the long axis of the tooth. These attachments require a well supported abutment tooth.

e.g. Dalbo 669.

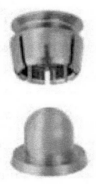

Dalbo 669 which is supplied in two sizes. There are 3 types of Dalbo attachments i.e. rigid, resilient and stress breaking type. The rigid Dalbo attachment has a cyclindrical male unit with a rounded head. The resilient attachment, the smallest and most commonly used of the types, allow vertical and horizontal movement of the female around a sphere shaped male unit made because of a relief space available between the unit while allowing some vertical movement of denture base before contact of male and female occurs.

Advantages of intra coronal over extra coronal retainers

1. They are more esthetic because retention is achieved through friction and not by visible retentive arms provided around the tooth contours.

2. They provide a more efficient cross arch stabilization of the abutment teeth.

3. They direct the vertical forces of occlusion along the long axis of the abutment teeth because rest seats are located within the normal contours of the abutment teeth and are closer to the horizontal axis of rotation.

4. The efficiency of retention is not affected by contours of abutment teeth

5. The number of components of denture is reduced and hence tolerance should be better.

6. When used with lower free end saddle, posterior movement is prevented

Disadvantages of intracoronal over extraocoronal retainers

1. They require placement of cast restoration on the abutment teeth which limits their use

2. They are effective in proportion of their length and are therefore least effective on short teeth and hence contraindicated for short teeth.

3. They should not be placed on teeth with large pulps because it might lead to pulp exposure.

4. They frequently tend to loosen during use because of frictional wear of the parts with subsequent removal with resultant loss of retention and increased torque stress on the teeth.

5. They require complicated clinical procedures and laboratory procedures

6. They are expensive and difficult to repair or even reline or rebase.

7. Intracoronal retainers are contraindicated in distal extension removable partial dentures unless an effective

types of stress breaking device is used between the denture base and the intra coronal retainer. A stress breaker is necessary to relieve the abutment teeth of all or part of the torquing stresses exerted on them by movable distal extension dentures.

CLASSIFICATIONS

I. ATTACHMENT CLASSIFICATION BY GOODKIND AND BAKER 1976

1. Intra coronal attachments

    a. Resilient intracoronal attachments (Resilient attachments allows movement to some degree)

    E.g. Crismani 689-A, Crismani 689-D.

    b. Non-resilient intracoronal attachments (Rigid attachments).

2. Extracoronal attachments

    a. Resilient extra-coronal attachments

    E.g. Crismani Resilience joint, Dalbo resilience joint.

    b. Non- resilient extra-coronal attachments

    E.g. Spang Stabilex, Spang Conex

II. ATTACHMENTS CAN BE CLASSIFIED DEPENDING ON WHETHER THEY ARE PRE-FABRICATED OR FABRICATED IN THE LABORATORY

1. Those pre-fabricated by the manufacturer is called as precision attachment.

    Pre-fabricated type of attachment is usually made of precious metal and are more precise than laboratory fabricated.[8]

2. Plastic attachments

    Simple, yet precise, indicated for removable and fixed denture.

III. PRECISION ATTACHMENTS CAN BE CLASSIFIED ACCORDING TO RIGID OR MOVABLE ARTICULATIONS (G.E.RAY)

a. **Rigid articulations :** (These are separable joints designed to prevent movement when fully articulated)

   Group I : Attachments used principally with vital teeth

   Group II : Anchorage used principally with pulp less teeth

b. **Moveable articulations :**

Group I : Conjunctors used principally with vital teeth

Group II : Conjunctors used principally with pulpless teeth

IV : PRECISION ATTACHMENTS ARE CLASSIFIED INTO :

(BY G.E. RAY)

a. Intracoronal attachment

b. Extracoronal attachment

c. Conjuctors

d. Anchors

e. Bars

f. Accessory components

Intracoronal attachments

They are very esthetic and provide cross arch stabilization.

Extracoronal attachments

Extracoronal attachments have two adavantages over Intracoronal designs:

1. They can be used without affecting the design of the preparation

2. They are not much of restrictions in its size and therefore can have greater freedom in designs

Therefore they can be fashioned to give greater retention and can include locking screws of latch type.

e.g. Stabilex extra coronal attachment

Flecher extra coronal attachment

Conjunctors

A conjunctor is a precision attachment made by the conjunction of an attachment to a stress breaker.

The primary role of a conjunctor is to permit movement between tissue borne and tooth borne.

Anchors

In fabrication of dentures or fixed restorations anchors are intended to provide retention and support for bars, partial denture and overdenture.

Wherever possible anchorage should be used with attachments, in order to relieve the soldered joints of the shear strain to which rigid designs are susceptible.

Anchors can be divided into those with ;

a. Screwed retention (Screw blocks)

b. Slide blocks

    1. Friction grip

    2. Snap grip

Screw-Block Anchors

They are of 3 basic types i.e. Hruska screw block are solid cores, notched, and tapped occlusally to accept small grub screws with tapered heads.

Schubiger system

Consists basically of a threaded post mounted on a circular soldering plate. A recessed collar slips over the post which is held in place by means of a cap nut that screws over the post to bear on an internal ledge within the collar. The collar can be either long or short. The collar is removable and used to provide fixation for a bar (by soldering the head of the bar to the collar) or can be provided with tagging for use within a bridge on an isolated crown. Short collar are used for usually for bars and long collars for crowns etc.

Harkowitsch System

Is based on one of two size of self tapping root canal posts which is used with a soft gold washer to hold a cemented root cap in place.

Slide block anchors

Slide block friction grip anchorage consist of circular posts which either enter a matrix cast within the diaphragm or when mounted on a soldering discs (for soldering to root raps) from patrices which enters a removable matrix.

Most friction grip slide block anchorage can be converted into resilient slide blocks by use of spacing washers which will permit a degree of vertical resilience

e.g. Gmur slide block anchor

Dalla Bona Slide block or Dalbostud anchor.

Snap grip slide blocks cannot be converted into resilience anchor because the active element locks into a predetermined groove but in other respects are similar to corresponding friction grip varieties.

Rothermann eccentric cylindrical snap grip anchor.

Huser anterior slide block anchor

Bars

Bars attchments are used for retention and support of removable bridges, removable partial dentures and overdentures. Their advantages lies in splinting action which they provide between isolated abutments.

Round, U shaped and ovoid bars are provided with tagged clips for processing within saddles.

e.g. U-shaped Dolder – Bar.

Accessory components

Accessory components include retentive elements, transverse stabilizers or locks, and stress breakers.

Example are :

Retention elements

a. Isoclip by Guigelmetti

Stress breakers

a. Strini hinge

b. Vertical cylindrical cone stress breaker

Transverse stabilizer or lock

a. Push lock designed by spang

b. Huser lock

V. PRECISION ATTACHMENT CAN BE DESCRIBED AS PASSIVE, ACTIVE, LOCKED (G.E. RAY)

Passive attachments

They are made in solid section so that patrix fits into the matrix in the fashion of interlocking parts of a jig saw, the retention between two parts depends on accuracy of the fits, shape of the joint, and area of contact.

e.g. Passive Omega attachment

Passive Beyler attachment

Active attachments

These attachments differ from passive attachments that some form of spring is used to give additional retention. Devices which incorporates leaf-springs, split rings or expanded collars are referred to Active friction grip attachments. They function by forcing part of the patrix against matrix, thereby increasing area of contact and effort required to separate them. The force exerted by these springs can be controlled by expanding the spring either with a razor blade of kit provided, hence these are also called as adjustable attachments.

Example of active friction grip attachments are Omega attachments active friction grip. McCollum attachment; active friction grip.

Another variety of active attachments use a spring loaded stud or split ring to engage in a prepared recess within the matrix so that the frictional retention is enhanced by a mechanical resistance to separation. When two halves of this type of joint complete their articulation the retention stud or ring snaps into groove or pit prepared for it, hence they are called as Active snap grip attachment. The tension of activat-ing spring of a snap-grip attachment can be altered. They are called also adjustable attachments.

Eg. Schatzmann Snap – Grip attachments

Locked precision attachments are either bolted together by means of a sliding bolt or latch (latch grip) or may by pinned or screwed together.

VI. PRECISION ATTACHMENTS HAVE BEEN CLASSIFIED ACCORDING TO ATTACHMENTS SHAPE. (HAROLD W. PREISKEL – PRECISION ATTACHMENTS IN DENTISTRY)

A. Intracoronal attachments

The two parts of an intracoronal attachments consists of a flange and a slot. The flange is joined to one section of the prosthesis and the slot unit is embedded in a restoration that forms another section of the prosthesis.

Two types of intracoronal attachments are available

a. Those whose retention is entirely frictional

E.g. The McCollum intra coronal unit.

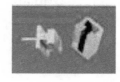

b. *Those whose retention is augmented by a mechanical lock.* Eg. The Schatzmann unit

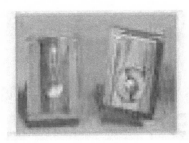

Additional retention is provided by a spring loaded plunger.

Depending on the cross sections intra coronal attachments (Harold W. Preiskel) can be classified into.

1. *H-Shaped flanges* (Most of the modern attachments have it and they have nearly double the frictional surface area. The external frictional flange of H-Shaped unit strengthen the attachment, without increasing the size of the female part.

2. *T-shaped flanges*

   Eg. The chayes attachment. This T-shaped unit is still in production today.

3. *Attachments with a circular cross section.* They are suitable only for joining two sections of a fixed prosthesis.

The friction fit intracoronal attachments with adjustment potential are :

e.g.

a. Chayes unit can adjusted by opening the two halves with a razor blade or scalpel.

b. The crismani series of intracoronal attachments

c. McCollum unit

d. Ancra attachment unit features a „H" shaped profile with external frictional flange while the male unit incorporates slots either side to allow for modification of retention.

e. The T-Geschiebe 123 has an external frictional flange cast together with a bracing arm

The attachments with auxillary retentive features :

Auxillary retentive features are incorporated in some attachments to provide more retention for a given frictional area.

a. The wide Crismani units incorporate a wire clip to increase retention. Access to the clip is obtained by removing the screw in the male unit. The female unit contains two depressions for retaining wire.

b. Some devices basically consists of a spring loaded piston on the male part engaging a socket within the female element like a simple cup board door catch.

E.g. Schatzmann attachment the retention of which is increased by a spring – loaded plunger assembly.

c. The Stern gingival latch attachment offers a novel method of additional retention. The base of the male unit is split and formed in the shape of a door latch. The result is to provide a lock as the male slide is engaged. Adjustments for retention are made with a purpose – built tool. Two sizes of unit are produced, standard and miniature. On the standard unit the splint is 2,5 mm and in the miniature unit it is 1.5 mm high.

d. Micro which is among the smallest of intracoronal attachments with auxillary includes a unit with squared lateral surfaces thereby allowing the bucco-lingual divergence to be reduced.

e. The Dovetail and ESI versions are modifications of the tagging of the male unit. The dovetail design simplified soldering. The ESI features a long extension plate that simplifies electrosoldering the male to the denture frame work. Alternatively the extension can be roughened to permit retention by the acrylic resin.

Before choosing an attachment with auxillary retentive devices the following factors should be considered.

- Bulk

- Adjustment

- Retention mechanism

- Trimming the attachment

- Plaque control

The friction fit intracoronal attachments without adjustment potential :

Lack of adjustment potential renders this type of unit unsuitable for removable prosthesis, as repeated insertion and removal will cause the attachment to wear. They are useful for joining a series of crowns without a common path of insertion. Round profiles are useful when anterior teeth are concerned.

e.g. Interlock attachment

Beyler attachment offers more frictional surfaces area and is used in posterior quadrants.

Applications of intracoronal attachments

1. **Retainers :** Intra coronal attachments are effective and almost invisible retainer for bilateral and unilateral prostheses.

2. **Connectors :** Sections of a fixed prosthesis may be joined together with intracoronal attachments. This possibility can be useful where;

   a. Prosthesis do not share a common path of insertion yet can be connected rigidly in the mouth.

b. The operator prefers to limit the length of individual castings while making a large span fixed prosthesis.

c. When the prognosis of a distal abutment is in doubt. Connecting the posterior segment with an attachment allows to subsequent removal without damage to the main restoration. The attachment slot can be used for later construction of an attachment retained denture

B. EXTRACORONAL ATTACHMENTS

These attachments have part or all of their mechanism outside the crown of a tooth. Many of these unit allow a certain amount of movement between the two sections of the prosthesis. Their main application is for distal extension prosthesis. They may be used to retain restorations for bounded spaces. Extracoronal attachments can be subdivided into following groups.

a. Projection units

The units are attached to the proximal surface of a crown. These groups can be divided in turn into;

1. Those that provide a rigid connection. Eg. Conex attach-
    ment (it has parallel walls that provide a precise patch of
    insertion)

2. Those that allow play between the components. Eg. Dalbo
    extracoronal projection unit, ceka system with retaining
    ring.

b. Connectors

These units connect two sections of a removable prosthesis and allow a certain degree of play.

Two basic types of joints are manufactured

1.   The axial rotation joint

It provides restricted vertical travel together with predetermined hinge movement. A small window is cut out of the
female section around the screw. The male section is therefore
free to travel up and down within the narrow confine of the
window. Rotation and lateral movements can be provided by
dismantling the attachment and very slightly trimming the
male unit. This joint can be incorporated within the Scott at-

tachment. Steiger originally envisaged the axial rotation joints as connector for distal extension denture.

2.   *The rotation joint*

Here there is no window around the screw and therefore vertical movements cannot take place. The rotation joint was designed for unilateral distal extension prosthesis as this type of denture is usually tooth and mucosal supported on one side and entirely tooth supported on the opposite side. Since vertical movement could be damaging to the teeth on the tooth supported side, Steiger designed the rotation joint to allow only slight rotational and lateral movements in order to minimize torque transmitted from the distal extension design would therefore incorporate an axial rotation joint connecting the distal extension base to the retainer and major connector, while the retainer on the opposite, tooth supported, side would be connected through a rotation joint. The Steiger joints are models of careful designs and are one of the few attachments in which the amount and direction of the movement allowance can be precisely determined by the operator. If appreciable wear takes place, both parts of the attachment can be removed from the mouth and a replacement soldered on. Boitel now finds that better results are obtained by using the rotation joint for bilateral distal extension base prosthesis as well.

C. *Stud attachment*

These attachments are so called because of the shape of the male units that are usually soldered to the diaphragm of a post crown. The female part fits over the male unit and is embedded within the acrylic resin of the prosthesis or soldered to a metal substructure.

There are a few systems in which the male section forms parts of the denture and the female part of the root surface preparation.

Few stud attachments are entirely rigid, since their size makes it difficult to prevent a small mount of movement between the two components.

In some attachments springs or other devices are specifically incorporated to allow a controlled degree of movement. Of all the stud attachments producd. Dalbo is by far the most popular. Although 3 types of design were produced the ball and socket design is most popular. It is smallest of the series it is 4 mm high. It allows limited vertical and rotational movement between the two parts of the attachment and has a spherical shaped male section that is easy to clean.

The rigid Dalbo attachment provides a firm connection between the two components but cannot match the versatility of the bal and socket unit.

The Battesti design are also of 3 designs. Two allow vertical translation of which one is ball and socket design. The third design is comparatively rigid.

Some of the other stud attachments available are Dr. Conod"s rigid stud unit, Rothermann unit, Baer and Fah units. Stud attachments have numerous applications to

1. *Overdenture* (being relatively small they can provide additional stability, retention and support while the positive lock of certain units can maintain the border seal of the denture).

2. *Non-vital parital denture abutments.* The loads applied in these circumstances can be considerable and for this rea-

sons, one of the larger and stronger, units is recommended.

3.   For retention of a small tooth supported restoration with non-vital abutment.

D. Bar Attachments

Bar attachments consists of a bar spanning an edentulous area joining together teeth or roots. The denture fits over the bar and is connected to it with one or more sleeves. Bar attachments are of 2 categories.

a. Bar joints

These units allow play between denture and bar. The bar is usually attached to diaphragms on root filled teeth, locking the roots together and improving the crown / root ratio. A common patch of insertion for the retaining posts is desirable although divergence can be overcome by mechanical means. Alternatively the abutment teeth can be crowned and these crowns connected by the bar.

Bar joints can be subdivided into :

1. Single sleeve bar joints

The Dolder bar joints is a good example of this attachment. This bar is produced from wrought wire, pear shaped in cross section and running just in contact with the oral mucosa between the abutments. An open sided sleeve is built into the impression surface of the denture and engages the bar when the denture is inserted.

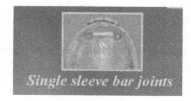

Single sleeve bar joints

Two sizes of Dolder bar joint are produced with heights of 3.5 mm and 4.5 mm. The cross sections are 2.3 mm x 1.6 mm and 3.00 mm x 2.2 mm, respectively. Apart from the artificial teeth, a sufficient bulk of acrylic resin must cover the sleeve to prevent fracture, although a lingual metal plate may be used when space is restricted. A spacer is provided with this bar joint to allow a degree of movement potential. The spacer is removed after the acrylic resin has been cured.

A bar joint that has become popular in the United states in known as Baker clip. It is available in 12 to 14 gauge bar size. The sleeve requires roughening to provide retention for the acrylic resin, no retentive tags are provided. The sleeve can be sectioned if the bar does not run in a straight line.

2. Multiple sleeve joints

If several short sleeves are substituted for the continuous one, there is no need for the bar to run straight and it can be bent to follow the vertical contours as well as the antero-posterior curvature of the ridges needed.

Gilmore"s original design was an attachment of this type and is still available today.

Ackerman"s bar is almost identical. It can be obtained in various shapes of across section. But it is the bar with circular cross section that tends to bend itself in all planes. As this unit has a small cross section and can be bent, it can frequently be positioned with a cleansable space under the bar, yet the bar does not interfere with positioning of the artificial teeth. The small sleeve units can be placed at most convenient sites.

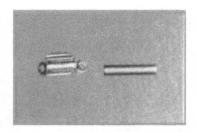

More rigid bar with pear shaped and oval cross sections are available, while a wax pattern of the bar is produced as well. This wax pattern can be contoured to correct shape and then cast in gold. The diameter needs reduction to about 1.8 mm after the casting process.

The Hader bar joint is provided by manufactures of pre-fabriciated plastic patterns that are adapated to the master cast and then cast in alloy of choice.

Multiple sleeve bar joints are more versatile than the single sleeve units, but the bars seem to have slightly less rigidity.

b. Bar units

Bar units are comparatively rigid allowing no movement between the sleeve and bar. Although some load may be distributed to the mucosa these prosthesis are mainly tooth borne. Bar units may be useful where;

1. There are 4 or more abutment teeth and large edentulous spaces.

2. The number of distribution of the teeth does not allow construction of a satisfactory clasp retained partial denture

3. These are edentulous areas with considerable resorption

4. Rigid splinting is required of the remaining teeth or roots.

5. The appearance of the remaining natural teeth requires post preparations

Bar units provide excellent retention and stability for a denture while rigidly splinting the abutments.[10] Artificial mucosa can be provided by the denture flange and the removable section can be rebased or repaired like a clasp retained prosthesis.

Drawbacks are that the bar provides a medium for accumulation of plaque and the patient must maintain a good standard of plaque control and denture hygiene.

Patients with poor manual dexterity cannot be expected to cope with such restorations. Other contraindications are those in which there is limited vertical or bucco lingual space.

Bar prosthesis are difficult to construct where heavy occlusal forces may be applied. There are also considerable technical difficulties in spanning a gap of more than 4 units with a bar unit owing to distortions that can occur.

The Dolder bar unit is a well established and reliable unit. The bar has parallel sides unlike the pear shaped profile of the bar joint. Retention for the sleeve is entirely frictional, provided by the parallel vertical surfaces of both sections.

E. AUXILLARY ATTACHMENT

This miscellaneous group consists basically of

a. *Screw units:*

These devices are useful for screwing and dismantling parts of a prosthesis in the mouth, when there is no common line of insertion of the whole. They are particularly useful for joining the two components of a telescopic crown.

Screw retained telescopic prosthesis : If the outer structure is retained by small screws, the prosthesis can act as an effective splint between the abutments, but still allows its removal by the dental surgeon.

Screw retaining for vital teeth: These components usually consists of a threaded sleeve of previous metal embedded within the inner copings, and a matched screw that passes through the outer section.

Eg. CM screw retaining systems available in different sizes and configurations

- HP screw and sleeve

Screw retaining for non-vital teeth: This system that has gained popularity consists of a previous metal block with a threaded screw hole attached to a post retained diaphragm. A removable section slides over the block and is screwed in position.

E.g. Hruska unit with two different sizes of block units available for anterior teeth together with a block unit suitable for posterior teeth.

The Schubiger screw system is extremely versatile, basically consisting of a threaded stud on base that can be soldered to a post diaphragm

b. Friction devices

Spring loaded plungers are commonly employed to increase retention between the two sections of a telescopic prosthesis E.g. Ipsoclip attachment. The spring loaded plunger mechan-ism may be dismantled by undoing, the bayonets clip at the opposite end of the plunger. The type of attachment is generally buried lingually in the outer, removable section of the prosthesis.

- Mini pressomatic unit. It is only 1.75 mm long, a small spring tensions the plunger.

Split posts : can be used in sectional dentures

E.g. P.W. Split post.

c. **Bolts**:

Bolts units are used to connect the two parts of sectional denture in the mouth. Each part of the denture is inserted separately and the patient locks them together with the bolt.

VII. CLASSIFICATION OF PRECISION ATTACHMENTS WHICH IS BASED ON THE USE OF WHICH THEY ARE PUT (DEVISED AT THE INSTITUTE OF DENTAL SURGERY, BY MR. R.VALENTINE IN COLLABORATION WITH COLLEAGUES, EASTMAN DENTAL HOSPITAL, LONDON).

Rigid retainers	- Rigid attachments (non vital teeth)	- Adjustable	- Chayes
			- McCollum
			- Stern
			- Crismani

		- Non-adjustable	- Beyeler
			-C&M643
- Rigid anchorages (on vital teeth)	- All adjustable	- Eccentric
			- Bona
			- Gerber

Movable retainers	- Movable attachments (Non vital teeth)	- Dalbo
		- Crismani
		- Gerber hinger
	- Stress breakers (for partial denture)	- Ancorvis hinger
		- Bona
	- Movable anchorages (non-vital teeth)	- Dolder bar
		- Andrews bar
Auxiliary devices		- Isoclip
	- Activators	- Schubiger
	- Latches, bolts, screws	- Hruska

VIII. ACCORDING TO TYPES OF INSTALLATION OF PRE-FABRICATION ATTACHMENT ON ABUTMENT CROWNS

a. *Intra coronal* Eg. McCollum attachment Schatzmann attachment

b. *Extra coronal or paracoronal*

c. *Interproximal attachment* E.g. Snaprox by Schatzmann

d. *Within a cantilevered bridge pontic* Eg. Biloc attachment with wraparound

e. *On a cantilevered pontic*

f. *Attachments in inter abutment bridge pontics*

g. *Prefabricated cap post systems on root copings* E.g. Gerber retention cylinder

MECHANISM OF ACTION

Retainers must hold the prosthesis securely in place during chewing swallowing, speaking and other oral functions. Therefore, male and female portions must fit together precisely.

Resistance to separation within the attachment is by following mechanisms.

1) **Friction :** Occurs when parallel walls of closely fitting bodies pass over one another.

Friction occurs between contacting parallel walled bodies. The frictional force is directly related to the area of the opposing surfaces as well as to the length of axial walls. The shape of the passage also plays a substantial role.

The holding ability of frictional attachment can be enhanced by addition of active retention elements.

> Spring – loaded bolts on plungers

> Leaf – springs

> Ring – springs

➤ Bolts

➤ Rubber devices

ii) **Binding** – Occurs when a parallel walled body tips within its receptor site.

Eccentric loads on frictional elements produce tipping movement, which create an additional binding effect significantly increasing resistance to withdrawal.

iii) **Wedging of conical bodies**

Friction comes into play only in the terminal position and is lost as soon as the bodies begin to separate.

iv) **Internal spring loading** as produced by a clip within a cylinder

The friction within retainers is often increased by loading with internal spring clips. Slots in the male portion allows the pressure to be adjusted.

v) **Active Retention**

That is when one body must be temporarily deformed to

be withdrawn from its fully seated position. Active retention means a physical obstruction to separation of other parts. One part must undergo elastic deformation before separation can occur.

Active retention by meant by means of a bulge at the end of a resilient slotted post. Active retention from a ring spacing.

ATTACHMENT SELECTION

In 1971, 126 attachment were listed and classified by Dr. Merrill Mensor, this is called as E. M. attachment selector.

It has 5 charts giving specification as to type, vertical dimension (Minimal and Maximal), whether it is for anterior and posterior teeth, whether the assembly is simple or complex, whether the function is rigid or resilient, type of resilience, size of movement and type of retention. It shows if the attachment is interchangeable or replaceable and finally what type of alloy and material it is made of.

E.M. attachment selector system utilizes a colour coded millimeter attachment gauge to define the vertical clearance available in the edentulous regions of occluded casts for attachment selection. The gauge is made of plastic and measuring 75 mm in length. It is graduated from 3 to 8 mm in 1 mm increments with a corresponding colour code. Red designates 3 to 4 mm, yellow designates 5 to 6 mm and black designates 7 to 8 mm. The gauge is placed between the occluded casts adjacent to a tooth that will carry an attachment. The measurement is thus read numerically and according to colour. The vertical limits measured by the EM gauge are the common area of concern for all connector systems. The available space will govern the type of attachment system that can be used. A closed vertical space will narrow the selection of available or recommended attachments. Where vertical inter-maxillary space is abundant, the choice of attachment systems is less restricting.

In selecting an attachment system;

i) **The first decision that must be made is whether to use an intracoronal attachment,**

ii) The second decision to be made is whether to use a resilient or a nonresilient type,

iii) The third consideration is that the largest attachment can be used within the given available space should be chosen to gain maximum stability, retention and strength for the prosthesis.

REQUIREMENTS OF PREFABRICATED AT-

TACHMENTS

The following requirements must be met:

1. Restoration of the masticatory apparatus to as optimum state of health

2. Consistent oral hygiene.

3. Periodontally suitable location of all elements of the prosthesis, and optimum cleansability.

4. Precise occlusal integration of all parts of the prosthesis into the patient"s individual neuromuscular pattern of function.

5. Suitable distribution of all retentive elements according to static and dynamic principles.

6. An equal degree of friction or active retention in all attachments (similarly designed elements)

7. Equal freedom of movement of all attachments.

8. A clearly defined path of insertion with simultaneous terminal stops of all attachments.

9. Rigidity of the entire prosthetic superstructure.

10. Adjustability or interchangeability of all frictional or actively retentive parts.

11. Possibility of modifying the structure to accommodate the loss of individual teeth (estimation of the risk).

12. Ability to reline all tooth-bearing denture bases.

INTRACORONAL VERSUS EXTRACORONAL ATTACHMENTS

The decision to an intracoronal or extracoronal attachment should be based on the size and shape the abutment teeth. Intracoronal attachments require more tooth preparation and tooth reduction than extracoronal attachments. If intracoronal attachment are used where there is insufficient space, the abutment retainer will be overcontoured on the proximal surface resulting in a restoration that can create periodontal problems.

When there is adequate space available, intracoronal attachments are preferred to extracoronal attachments. Because intracoronal attachments more ideally direct the forces of function along the long axis of abutment teeth.when there is inadequate space, an extacoronal prosthesis may be employed. However, the effects of extracoronal attachments might not be overlooked. The lever arm associated with the extracoronal attachment has the potential to direct forces that are not always directed along the long axis of the direct retainer. In addition, these extensions can create difficult areas for the patient in maintaining the health of the subjacent gingival tissues.

Resilient versus non-resilient attachments

The primary determining factor whether to use a resilient or non-resilient attachment has to do with personal preferences based on educational and clinical experiences. Resilient attachments allow for a predetermined amount of movement between abutment retainers and removable partial denture during function. The non resilient attachments are rigid non functioning attachments.

The major difference of philosophy regarding the use between two attachment occurs when dealing with distal extension edentulous situations (Kennedy Class I and Class II). Theoretically, the resilient attachment allows the functional forces to be directed to the tissue and alveolar ridge and the non-resilient attachment primarily directs the vertical functional forces to the abutment teeth. Realistically there is some sharing of the functional load in both systems.

In distal extension situations, where rigid intracoronal attachment are being used, splinting of the abutment teeth is recommended.

The least complicated attachments are usually considered most practical for use when all other factors are considered. Where adequate retention can be obtained with a simple frictional intracoronal attachment, its use is desired over a more complex system.

PRECISION ATTACHMENTS IN OVER-

DENTURES

F. Attachment Fixation Overdenture

The overdenture may connect to the copings with studs or other attachment bar-and-rider systems.

Indications

1. Roots are retained for conservation of the alveolar ridge.

2. Over denture support, stability and retention are all important considerations.

3. Coping coverage is indicated for caries control.

4. Weak abutments require splinting (though some attachments can be utilized without splinting the roots).

5. The dentist desires controlled adjustable retention.

6. Comfort and patient acceptance are major concerns. (An attachment-retained overdenture feels more like bridge work than a non-attachment overdenture.)

7. The dentist wishes to minimize, or maximize, the amount of denture-bearing mucosa.

8. The dentist desires a more balanced distribution of masticatory load between abutments and tissue than is possible with a conventional telescopic overdenture.

Disadvantage

1. **More expensive than conventional telescopic overdenture.**

2. More difficult to fabricate.

3. More difficult to maintain.

4. Some attachments are bulky and therefore may cause esthetic and occlusal space problems.

5. Patients with limited manual dexterity may have difficulty inserting the prosthesis.

Superiority of Attachment-Fixation Overdenture

The attachment-fixation overdenture is far superior to other types of overdentures or other forms of overlay prostheses. It can more closely approximate the results obtained with fixed dridgework and precision partial denture prosthetics than is possible with telescopic overdentures complete dentures. The patient is more secure in its use than with a complete denture. Thus, he enjoys increased comfort, function, and a more natural appearance.

Whether an extra-coronal or intra-coronal attachment is to be utilized, the dentist must make his selection based upon his knowledge of such factors as a) crown-root ratio desired, b) type of copings, c)vertical space available, d) number of teeth present, e) amount of bone support, f) location of abutments, and h) whether the overdenture is to be a tooth-supported **or** a i) tooth-tissue-supported appliance. In addition, such factors as the type of j) opposing dentition is important, for example, whether a complete denture, overdenture, or natural dentition k) maintenance problems and, of least importance, the 1) cost. These selection principles will be considered in detail when discussing the specific attachment

Resilient or Non-Resilient Attachments

Many of the most popular attachments are available in both resilient and non-resilient designs. This is a mechanism for controlling distribution of the forces of masti-

cation uniformly over the denture-bearing mucosa and the supporting abutments. Attachments should be selected on the basis of this action.

1. A resilient attachment reduces vertical and lateral forces on the abutments by distributing more of the masticatory load to the tissues. This is accomplished by fabrication a gap of 0.5-1 millimeter between the overdenture and the metal substructure. When the denture is out of function, it rests entirely on the mucosa. Only during function (after the tissues have compressed 0.5-1 millimeter) are vertical forces transmitted to the sub-structure and thus to the roots. Resiliency is a special advantage when the denture base fits poorly due to alveolar resorption, faulty fabrication, an inadequately fitted denture base, or errors in cementation of the substructure (the space helps to accommodate the above errors in fit).

Use resilient attachments

a) For a tissue-tooth supported appliance.

b) With very weak abutments, when maximum tissue support

is required.

c) When there are only a few abutments.

d) When functioning opposite natural dentition.

e) When functioning against a non-resilient appliance.

f) When multi-directional action is desired.

g) With minimal denture base.

2. A non-resilient attachment, as its name implies, does not permit any vertical movement during function. If the appliance is entirely tooth-supported, the abutments must withstand the entire masticatory load.

Of course, if the prosthesis rests on the abutments and mucosa at the same time, then the mucosa also supports some of the load during function. An attachment having some rotational movement should be used in such a situation. It compensates for some of the functional loading on the abutments by directing some of these forces to the supporting mucosa.

This maximal loading is less stressful to non-resilient

restored abutments when the denture base is broadened and well adapted to the supporting mucosa.

Use non-resilient attachments

a) When no vertical movement is indicated, but where rotational action may be desirable.

b) With an all-tooth support appliance.

c) With a tooth-tissue-supported appliance.

d) With strong abutments.

e) When functioning against a complete denture.

f) When functioning against a resilient overdenture.

g) When large, well-fitting denture base

h) Where intra-occlusal space is limited.

Uses of general types of precision attachments

1. Bar attachments

a) For splinting abutments.

b) For retention, stability and support.

c) Where adequate vertical space is available.

d) Can be used with all coping sizes.

e) Personal preference.

2. *Stud attachments*

a) For retention, stability and support,

b) Where vertical space is limited (depends upon selection of specific stud).

c) Used generally with short copings.

d) Can be positioned strategically along a splinted span of abutments.

e) For maximum tissue support.

f) Personal preference.

3. *Auxiliary attachments*

a) Spring-loaded plunger attachment

For retention only. Generally used to engage the side of long or medium copings. May be used for retention with bars. Personal preferences.

b) screws

For firm fixation. For fixation with another attachment system.

For specialized conditions

Bar Attachment Selection

An important feature of the bar attachment is its rigid splinting of the abutments. However, it requires more space vertically, facially and lingually than a stud attachment. There are two basic types of bar attachments based on their shape and action provided. For example: 1. Bar Unit and 2. Bar joint.

1. *Factors to be Considered for Bar Selection*

Bar Unit-As the name implies, it acts as a fixed unit. This bar has parallel walls providing rigid fixation with frictional retention. Due to the shape of the bar there will be on rotational or vertical movement of the overlay prosthesis.

This attachment can be used with long, medium or short copings, but only when this appliance is to be tooth supported and no stress-broken action is indicated. It is never used where a bar joint (a movable action) is indicated.

However, a bar joint can be used as a substitute for the bar unit; when the bar joint is not spaced, and when the prosthesis is tooth supported.

Bar joint-It has a curved contour, which permits the prosthesis to rotate around the bar slightly. This action minimizes the torquing of the bar (and, of course, the roots) during mastication ad allows the tissues to assume some of the load. The bar joint may also feature vertical movement with the prosthesis. Since the typical overdenture case involves weak abutments, the more gentle bar joint is preferred to the rigid modification.

It is a vary useful attachment when used

a) Provides vertical and /or rotational action.

b) For retention, support and stability.

c) For splinting abutments.

d) Used with short copings.

e) Used with short copings.

f) Available as resilient.

g) Contraindicated with minimal intra occlusal space.

2. Number of bar attachments that are applicable for removable prosthesis.

a) Dolder bar

b) Hader bar

c) Andrews bar

d) Ceka

e) Octalink

f) C.M. bar

g) M. P. Channels

h) Ackerman bar

i) Customized bars

G. *Stud Attachment Selection*

A large variety of stud attachments are available for overdenture use. Most consist of a post-like male secured to the diaphragm of the coping. The female which engages the male post is processed within the tissue side of the denture. These components engage each other when the overdenture is inserted. Generally, the retention is obtained by a frictional fit of the female on the male, or a "snap-like" action when the female engages an undercut on the male. Most stud attachments are available as non-resilient or as resilient attachments.

1.   *Factors to be Considered for Stud Selection*

Consider these features when selecting a stud attachment:

a) Can be used on single copings.

b) Can be positioned strategically on a coping splint.

c) May have a much narrower and lower profile. This means that a stud: may be used with a short coping for a very favorable space; permits a highly esthetic overdenture due to its narrow width.

d) Available in a wide variety of designs from simple to complex.

e) Available as non-resilient or resilient varieties.

f) Produces the least bulky overdenture.

g) For retention, stability and support.

h) Limited in its use on very weak, nonsplinted single abutments.

i) Can allow denture movement in several directions.

j) Personal preference.

2. Here are few examples of some common stud attachments:

a) Dalla Bona

b) Gerber

c) Ceka

d) Rothermannn

e) Gmur

f) Huser

g) Schubiger

h) Ancrofix

Auxiliary Attachment Selection

Auxiliary attachments are in the category of specialized screws, or spring-loaded plunger types of attachments.

Pressure-button attachments such as the Ipsoclip and IC types have a spring-loaded plunger. This plunger engages a small depression prepared within the coping or surface of a bar. They can provide auxiliary retention with long or medium copings or bars. They are used only where no rotational movement is programmed into the appliance, although they can be used where vertical resilience is present. therefore they are often used where abutment teeth are present in more than one plane. The selection of a specific pressure-button attachment would be based upon the characteristics of the particular attachment.

1. Features of Plunger-type attachment

These are some characteristics of the plunger attachment:

a) Can engage long and medium copings to retain a telscopic overdenture.

b) Can be used to engage bars for retention.

c) Some are self-contained or have replaceable parts.

d) Some can be processed in the acrylic resin denture base, soldered or cast into the secondary coping of an overdenture.

e) May be used to add additional retention to an already existing overlay prosthesis.

2. Plunger-type attachment.

Listed below are a few of the plunger-type attachments:

a) Ipsoclip

b) Pressomatic

c) IC attachment

Of these, the IC attachment is simple in design and low I cost.

3.   Auxiliary Screw Attachment Selection

Screws have a rather limited use in overdenture prosthetics, but can become an invaluable adjunct to attachments in special situations. Screw attachments contribute a fixed removable characteristic to an overlay prosthesis and permit easier modification of the prosthesis.

Screws may be used for fixation of removable bridgework, for attachment of bars to stud posts and as anchor attachments for individual crowns. Screws would be considered under the following conditions.

1. Fixation with fixed-removable bridge-work

2. For individual crown anchorage.

3. For splinting bars to studded copings on divergent teeth.

4. With a bar prosthesis, where the bar can be removed for easy modification.

5. Personal preference.

4. **Screw attachments**

The selection of screws is rather limited. Of all the screws, the Schubiger attachment is most widely used in overdenture prosthetics. It is used under most conditions mentioned above, with the exception of single-crown anchorage, and will be considered in more detail later in this text.

The VK-screw system can be used for the fixation of primary copings to roots, or fixation of secondary copings or bars to the supporting abutments.

PREFABRICATED PRECISION ATTACHMENTS

ZEST ANCHOR

Simple root-supported overdentures can be made more effective by incorporating an Intracoronal root attachment such as the Zest anchor.

The attachment

The Zest anchor is an ideal attachment for use with an overlay prostheses to provide retention and support. The fact that this particular attachment can be used with or without copings makes it an ideal attachment when economy or an intermediate treatment plan is a consideration.

This attachment system has numerous components female, white male post with spacer, blue transfer post with spacer, support cap, red substitute female, ceramic rod with female, sizing drill and number forty two drill.

Advantages

1. Overcomes any space problem because attachment is within root structure.

2. Leverage on the abutment tooth is negligible, since the part of attachment is well below alveolar bone level.

3. The attachment procedure is simple, can be performed quickly at chair side and can be done without any casting.

4. In cases where more than one tooth is used parallelism is not necessary because of the flexibility of the nylon male.

Disadvantage

1. Susceptible to caries since on casting or coping is made over the root structure.

2. Nylon studs can be dent, preventing seating of the application especially if several are use or they might even fracture.

3. Food lodgment in the female housing if patient attempts eating without denture in place.

Attachment Function

The female is cemented within a special recess prepared inside the occlusal portion of a non-vital root with a special sizing bur. The nylon male, which provides retention, is processed within the tissue side of the over denture. Positive retention and support are accomplished when the terminal bell portion of the male engages the internal undercut of the female when the denture is inserted.

Zest Anchor Components

Listed below are various Zest components.

1. **Diamond sizing bur.** This special diamond bur is used to prepare a recess in the root to receive the female portion of the Zest anchor. It is available for a standard female and mini-female. It is also available to fit either a latch-type or a friction-grip handpiece.

2. **Female.** This portion of the attachment, which is cemented in the prepared root, is available in standard size, for large roots and in a mini-size for smaller roots.

3. **White nylon male.** This male post is processed in the tissue side of the denture base. It engages the female undercut when the overdenture is inserted.

4. **Male centering sleeve.** The male centering sleeve fits over the male post and aids in accurately positioning the male inside the female during fabrication for effective retention.

5. **Support cap.** The support cap permits the dentist to fit a root with a female, yet not activate it for retention. Since it has no terminal ball, it only provides vertical and lateral support to the denture over lay.

6. **Blue transfer male.** This simulated male with its centering sleeve, is used during relining procedures, or during original fabrication when using the indirect technique for positioning the white male post inside the denture. Its diameter is smaller then that of an actual male (the white male post). Therefore it is more easily removed with the master impression. The transfer male is discarded after denture fabrication.

7. **Red substitute female.** Used with the blue transfer males for the techniques described above.

8. **Male spacer.** Used to create a space within the denture base, so the regular male post can be picked up directly in the mouth using self-curing resin.

9. **Ceramic rod with female attachment.** This assembly is used to place a metal female into the wax coping pattern to produce a gold casting with a metal female.

10. **Number forty two drill.** Used to make a hole in the middle of the root on the master cast to receive a male spacer. This

technique is used when the male is to the positioned directly on the denture in the mouth.

Basic techniques

There are two basic techniques for managing the patient with
a Zest anchored overdenture

a. The indirect approach involves the prior positioning of
the females into endodontically treated teeth. Then
transfer males are placed into the females and a master
impression is taken of the denture bearing areas and the
roots with the females fitted with transfer males. The
transfer males are withdrawn with the impression, and
females snapped over the posts so that a master cast is
produced with substitute females accurately positioned
on the cast. The overlay prosthesis is fabricated on the
casts in such a way that the males become accurately
fabricated in the denture base.

b. The direct approach involves the prior fabrication of the
overlay prosthesis without males. After the overlay prosthesis is delivered to the dentist, the endodontically

treated teeth are fitted with the females. The males are then locked into special recesses within the denture directly in the mouth with self curing resin.

Indirect procedure

Steps in the indirect procedure

1. Examination, diagnosis, treatment plan

2. Periodontal therapy and endodontics

3. Prepare the roots

4. Insert females into roots

5. Place transfer male into cemented females

6. Take master impression for the overlay prosthesis with the withdrawn transfer males in position

7. Place red substitute females or, preferably, regular females over the males in the impression

8. Pour impression to produce cast with transfer females locked in position.

9. Take occlusal registration

10. Set up and articulate teeth

11. Place white males on the cast inside the females

12. Process overlay prosthesis with males in place

Root preparation and seating of females

1. For this treatment all periodontal therapy and extractions should be completed several months prior to the initial operative appointment

2. Use a high speed handpiece with a carbide fissure bur to reduce the teeth to approximately 3-4 mm above the gingival tissues initially

3. If endodontics had not been previously completed, it may be accomplished at this time. Such treatment is greatly simplified by the prior removal of the crown and reduction of the root. With improved access to the canal of the tooth, the canal can be mechanically manipulated with a reduction gear contra angle and appropriate drills, a special contra angle with latch type reamers, or with hand instrumentation. Only the apical portion of the root is filled to allow adequate room for the post of the female.

4. Each root surface is now reduced with a diamond bur in the same plane slightly above the gingiva. This adjustment cut is made at right angles to the path of insertion of the overdenture (in relation to soft tissue undercuts and the pulp canal of each tooth). When making this cut, or reduction, stop when 0.5 to 1.0 millimeter from the gingiva (at its nearest point). This produces the most favorable crown – root ratio, with little danger of the female being below the gingival creast. Remember, the root surface must be high enough o permit a round periphery. The cut and contoured surface should not be submerged bellow the gingiva. Other wise, the gingiva will proliferate over the abutments.

5. To prepare a recess into the canal drill a six millimeter pilot hole into the canal with a number two round bur. Drill these pilot holes parallel to each other and to the path of insertion. When making the pilot holes where the females are not to follow the root canal, due to differences in the path of insertion and because of the soft tissue and bone undercuts, care should be exercised so as not

to perforate the root wall. When preparing recesses in multiple rooted teeth, do not perforate the pulpal floor.

6. Next, enlarge the occlusal three to four millimeters of the pilot hole with a fissure or number six round bur to a size slightly smaller than the main body of the female. This eliminates excess drilling with the sizing bur.

7. Prepare the female recess with the special diamond sizing bur. It is best to use a reduction gear contra angle at a slow speed to avoid excessive movement that might over size the recess, or even break the post portion of the drill. If the opening is inadvertently made too large so the female does not fit snugly, fill the recess with amalgam or a composite filling material and re-prepare. If the canal cannot be followed, remove both the post portion of the drill and the female, or use the mini drill and mini female. The hole should be drilled so that a very, very slight recess is also created on the occlusal root surface with the disc portion of the drill. The female will fit into this recess like an inlay.

8. The female are now ready to the cemented into the roots. Mix, the crown and bridge cement to the proper consistency for cementing an inlay. Introduce cement deep into the recess with a lentulospiral drill. Next, insert a male attachment into the female with the centering sleeve in position. Add cements to the female, and using the inserted male as a handle, insert the female into the recess. Keep firm pressure on the male until initial set of the cement.

9. After final set of the cement, remove the male post and all excess cement.

10. The root surface is now ready for final preparation and finishing. With a fine diamond bur, remove all sharp corners at the root periphery. Contour, shape and drill toward the gingival margin, but end this contour and root margin approximately 0.5 millimeter above the gingiva. Finally, polish the root surface with appropriate discs and rubber wheels.

Indirect procedure for processing males into the denture

1. After females have been cemented into the roots, the blue transfer posts, with their centering sleeves, are now inserted into the females in each root. These male posts have slightly less retention than that of the white males, and will be withdrawn easily with the impression.

2. On a previously fabricated study cast, construct a custom tray for a mater impression. Drill holes through the tray over the area of the male posts. These holes minimize possible distortion or dislodgment of the male transfer posts.

3. Since the teeth are reduced to the gingival crest, eh arch can be treated as if it were edentulous. Therefore, the tray is muscle trimmed with molding compound to produce an accurate record of the peripheral soft tissue attachments. A master impression may be taken with a zinc oxide impression paste; or even rubber base impression material. Record the denture bearing ridge area and

the roots with their females. The transfer posts are then withdrawn within the impression material. This impression can be made with the impression material of your choice.

4. When the impression is removed, you will notice the ends of the male posts extending out of the impression material. Place spare females or the red substitute females over the ends of these transfer males. These females must be snapped firmly over the posts, but with care so as not to dislodge the males.

5. Pour the cast using the impression, with the transfer females locked securely in place. The transfer females now become an integral part of the master cast (representing the females in the patient"s mouth.

6. The master cast for the fabrication of the overdenture is now completed.

7. This master cast is used to fabricate a occlusal tray with wax rims for occlusal registration. This occlusal tray may

be a shellac tray, a tray made of self curing resin, or even the metal framework used as part of the final prosthesis.

8. For added retention and stability when you take occlusal records, the tray may be fitted with the white. Zest males. To do this, place a hole in the tray over each transfer female to receive the white male posts. Lock the male to the tray or metal framework, with a hard wax or selfcuring resin. Use of the white males during occlusal registration also aids in the set-up of the denture teeth.

9. Occlusal records are now taken with the technique of your choice.

10. The occlusal records are used to articulate the casts on an appropriate articulator.

11. Before set up of the denture teeth, insert the white male firmly into each female. Push down each centering sleeve to accurately position each male. This makes the ball of the male firmly engage the female undercut for maximum retention.

12. Bock out all undercuts around the roots with plaster.

13. Set up the denture teeth. The denture set up is then checked in the mouth for occlusion and any esthetic modification.

14. Wax, festoon, flask, pack and finish as you would any conventional complete denture

15. Remove the centering sleeve and excess flash from around each male post. The overdenture is now ready for insertion.

Direct technique

In the direct technique, the overdenture is first fabricated without the Zest males. The females are placed into the abutments, the males snapped into the females, and then locked directly into the overdenture in the mouth. The recess inside the overdenture to receive the males either can be prepared chairside by the dentist, or processes into the overdenture using special male spacers. The following procedure describes the direct technique using male spacers to prepare a recess inside the overdenture to receive the male directly in the mouth.

---

1. Using the procedure of your choice, take a master impression of the denture bearing ridge areas and existing dentition. The resulting cast will be treated similar to that for an immediate denture insertion.

2. Fabricate custom trays for recording the occlusal registration. Mount the casts on an appropriate articulator.

3. Trim the teeth on the cast to simulate the reduced abutments. Remove the teeth on the cast that are to be extracted later.

4. Using a number forty two drill in a straight handpiece, prepare a hole in the cast of each root that will be fitted with a Zest female. Following the long axis of each tooth, drill the holes parallel to the path of insertion.

5. Insert the special red male spacers into these holes. The spacers assist in the setup of the teeth by providing adequate room for the nylon male. If the holes are drilled correctly, the male spacers should be in correct position over each root. The spacers will be removed after the overdenture is processed, leaving a recess in the

tissue side of the denture to accommodate the hub of the white male. You may make adjustments to these recesses, or to the nylon male, if necessary.

6. Set up the denture teeth, articulate, wax, and festoon as you would a conventional complete denture.

7. The denture is half flasked, full-flasked, processed and polished with the spacer in place.

8. Remove the male spacers leaving recesses within the overdenture base to receive the male posts. The overdenture is now delivered to the dentist for insertion.

9. Now the teeth must be prepared to receive the Zest females. The endodontically treated teeth are prepared to receive the females as described earlier. The females are cemented and the denture is ready for insertion and positioning of the male posts.

10. Any teeth to be removed should be extracted at this time.

11. Next, test the fit of the overdenture to be certain that it sits passively on the tissues when it is in position. If any

rocking is present, remove any denture material that may be impinging upon the prepared roots or the females.

12. Place a small amount of Vaseline into the females before inserting the males. This prevents self curing resin from getting into the females. Snap the white nylon male, with its centering sleeve, into the cemented female until a definite snap is felt. The centering sleeve must be firmly seated into the female. This sleeve serves to position the male in proper alignment to engage the female under cut and prevents acrylic resin from entering the female.

13. Insert the denture to be certain it sits passively over the male hub. If it does not, trim the hub or enlarge the male recess inside the overdenture until it does sit passively.

14. Remove the denture. With a small brush paint a small amount of self curing acrylic resin around and particularly under the protruding male hub.

15. Place a small amount of resin into the recess in the tissue side of the overdenture

16. Carefully insert the denture into position. The patient should be instructed to gently close into occlusion and to hold this position until the acrylic resin hardens. Thus, the male is processed in place by the self curing resin with the denture in occlusion.

17. After the acrylic has cured, remove the overdenture, trim excess flash, and remove the centering sleeves. The overdenture is now ready for use.

MINI ZEST ANCHORAGE

The mini zest is smaller than the regular Zest, being approximately 3.25 millimeters in length. Because of this, it is often more applicable in the following situations.

1. It should be used with smaller diameter roots, such as upper laterals, some bicuspids roots, lower anteriors, and in the pulp chamber of multi rooted teeth.

2. It may also be used when the pulpal chamber of teeth is very divergent from the path of insertion.

RELINING AND REABASING PROCEDURS

Torquing will cause severe damage to the remaining supporting abutments, if the problem is not corrected. Unstable overdentures must be relined or rebased.

1. If severe undercuts are present in the overdenture, trim the inside of the denture flange sufficiently to remove these undercuts.

2. Remove all male attachments and ream out additional denture base to provide room from impression material and new Zest males.

3. Place blue transfer posts into the females. The males should be accurately positioned with the centering sleeves, as described earlier.

4. Reposition the denture in the mouth to assure that the denture sits passively over the male posts. If not, remove additional acrylic resin over each post, or trim the hub of the males.

5. Remove the denture, dry it thoroughly and then paint an adhesive material inside the overdenture. Take a relining impression with the material of your choice. Have the patient ease gently into occlusion as you border mold the denture by muscle trimming.

6. When the impression material sets, remove the denture. The male posts will be retained within the impression material.

7. Place transfer females over each male

8. Pour the impression with stone material and trim the hard cast base

9. Accurately mount the cast with the retained overdenture in a relining jig, as you would any conventional relining procedure. Separate the relining jig, leaving the incisal and occlusal teeth imprint in the upper member, and the cast on the lower member.

10. Remove the cast from the jig and pry off the overdenture. Remove the denture teeth and insert them in their respective plaster indexes.

11. Place white Zest males into the transfer females locked in the master model. Position the centering sleeve and block out all root undercuts with plaster.

12. Reposition the cast on the relining jig and close the jig with the teeth in position. Trim the male hub if it hits against any denture teeth. Wax the teeth into position. Wax up the denture base and complete the overdenture, as described earlier.

13. The rebased denture is now ready for insertion.

Replacement of broken male posts

Often when the soft or bony tissue undercuts are excessive, it is difficult for the patient to accurately insert the overdenture. Here, insertion will cause excessive flexing of the male and thus encourage breakage. Occasionally the patient will develop a habit of biting the overdenture in place. This is a bad habit since the chances of breaking male posts are increased.

Excessive breakage, or premature wear of the male posts, is usually due to specific causes; for example ; poor occlusion, over extended denture flanges misaligned females, an inaccurately fitting overdenture, or where the alveolar process has resorbed excessively. Replacing the male posts should not be done without correcting the cause of the excessive wear; otherwise, breakage will continue.

Replacing the males

1. Remove the male post from the denture base. Remove additional acrylic to provide room for the new male post.

2. Insert a white male into the female

3. Inset the overdenture to be sure that it fits passively over the male.

4. Remove the overdenture and the male post

5. Place a small amount of Vaseline into the female, insert the male firmly into place. Align the male by firmly seating the centering sleeve. Then remove any excess Vaseline.

6. Place a small amount of self curing resin around and under the hub of the male post and a minimal amount into the over denture recess.

7. Insert the overdenture and have the patient close lightly into occlusion until the acrylic resin cures

8. remove the overdenture from the mouth. Remove the centering sleeve and any excess acrylic flash. The over-denture is now ready for insertion.

TROUBLE SHOOTING WITH ZEST ANCHOR

The Zest also may be used directly with previously con-structed copings where other attachments have failed under an overdenture. To trouble shoot such a failure with a Zest anchor, follow these procedures.

1. Drill pilot holes through the castings with a number four round bur being careful not to drill into the root. Contin-ue with a number two round bur into the root, approx-imately six millimeters

2. Enlarge the hole in the casting with a carbide fissure bur to receive the diamond sizing bur

3. Use the carbide fissure bur to flatten and parallel the occlusal surface of the copings to receive the flat area of the diamond but. This will minimize the drilling that is necessary with the diamond sizing bur to produce the female recess.

4. cement the female into the casting as you would an inlay. The Zest anchor will also provide retention for the coping, acting as a post.

5. Insert the nylon males into the females and process into the previously constructed as described earlier.

Stud attachments

Stud anchorage systems are particularly useful as retainers for overlay prostheses. They are versatile in design and application.

Studs are generally used on short copings, where they may be mounted on independent abutments or placed strategically along a span of splinted abutments. A wide variety of studs are available, permitting the dentist to limit and redirect the maximal loading on the mucosa and the abutments.

A stud may be resilient (and thus permit a slight vertical movement) or non resilient. Both resilient and non resilient studs may also offer "hinge freedom" in which the prosthesis rotates much like a bar joint.

Stud attachments may be considered for some of the following conditions

1. For retention, stability and support for an overlay prosthesis.

2. On individual short copings with adequate bone support

3. On individual short copings too distant from each other for use with bars.

4. For strategic placement on a splinted span of short copings

5. For strategic placement on splinted copings when a loss of an abutment is anticipated

6. Where vertical space is limited

7. For maximum esthetics, not possible with most bar systems

8. For maximum tissue support

9. For use with copings under the denture bases of partial dentures

10. Personal preference

Use of Resilient Stud

A resilient attachment permits the tissue to compress slightly before any load is transmitted to the abutment. It is usually preferred.

1. When there are only a few abutments

2. When abutments have minimal bone support

3. For tissue tooth supported prosthesis

4. When functioning opposite natural dentition

5. When functioning against a non resilient appliance (do not use opposite another resilient appliance).

6. When multi directional (stress broken) action is desirable

7. When there is a minimum denture base

8. To compensate for tissue resorption, ill fitting prosthesis, or errors in substructure cementation

Use Non Resilient Stud Attachment

A non resilient attachment will not allow vertical movement (however, it may permit rotation). It is preferred.

1. When no vertical movement is indicated

2. When an all tooth supported prosthesis is desired

3. When a tooth tissue supported appliance is desired

4. With strong abutments having maximum bone support (one half or more).

5. When functioning against a resilient prosthesis

6. When a large, well fitting denture base is possible

7. When there is little interocclusal space

8. Opposite a complete denture

Other stud attachments

1. Dalla Bona

2. Introfix

3. Ancrofix

4. Gerber

5. Gmur

6. rotehrmannn

7. Huser

8. Schubiger

9. Ceka

The Gerber attachments and its functions

The Gerber stud system is a versatile stud attachment used routinely. It consists of a male post soldered to the coping and a retentive female secured within the denture base of the overlay prosthesis. The Gerber attachment is furnished into two different types – a resilient and non resilient form. The male post consist of two parts –a threaded base, which is soldered to the diaphragm of a coping, a removable sleeve with a retentive undercut. The resilient female consists of a female housing copper shim, coil spring, a spring retaining sleeve, C-spring, and threaded retainer. The non resilient female has no copper shim, spring coil or spring retaining sleeve. Convenient tools are also used in the fabrication – female screw driver, male screw driver, paralleling mandrel, heating bar, and a soldering cornal.

Clinical and Technical procedures

1. Examination, study casts, diagnosis, treatment planning

2. Prophylaxis, soft tissue curettage, home care instructions

3. Fabrication of interim overdenture on study casts

4. Reduction of clinical crowns

5. Initial endodontic therapy (may be completed)

6. Extractions

7. Completion of periodontal therapy

8. Insertion of interim overdentures

9. Final endodontic therapy (if not completed)

10. Operative appointments

11. Laboratory procedures

12. Insertion of prosthesis

Non-resilient Gerber

The non-resilient Gerber attachment technique is similar to that described above but with one exception. As it is non-resilient, the overdenture and female rest on the tissues, copings and male posts in a passive position, no spacing is necessary.

Advantages of the Gerber attachment

1. It provides adequate retention, stability and support

2. Its retention is light and easily adjustable with springs adjustable and readily replaced

3. All of its post sleeves are interchangeable and replaceable, with the exception of the male screw base.

4. It can be used in conjunction with bars, especially when used with the Schubiger screw base.

5. It can be processed directly into the overdenture or positioned in the mouth with auto-polymerizing resin.

Disadvantages of Gerber attachment

1. It is a complex attachment and maintenance problems are relatively common. The male sleeve may become loose. The internal parts of the female may dislodge when the retaining screw unthreads.

2. Its large vertical dimension makes it impractical for minimal intraocclusal space

3. It requires an assortment of tools for fabrication and maintenance

4. The attachments must be parallel

5. The Gerber permits very little rotational action, so torquing of abutment teeth will occur with alveolar resorption.

DALLA BONA ATTACHMENT

Dalla Bona is a simple stud attachment making an excellent overdenture attachment, available in a resilient or non-resilient series. It is useful when there is minimal vertical space and where rotation, resilience and retention are desired.

It consists of a single piece male stud soldered to the coping and a single unit female processed within the denture. It is available in two types : cylindrical and spherical. One form even has an internal coiled spring much like the resilient Gerber. This spring much like the resilient Gerber. This Spring helps control vertical movement.

1. Cylindrical Dalla Bona

The cylindrical male post has parallel walls without an undercut. The female lamella fits snugly over the male posts, providing frictional retention. A PVC ring fits around the female lamellae. This aids in fabrication, and permits the lamellae to flex. The cylindrical Dalla Bona must be parallel, therefore, the male posts must be assembled using a paralleling mandrel and suveyor.

2. Spherical Dalla Bona

The spherical Dalla Bona is similar to the cylindrical, but the male post is spherical. This sphere provides a retentive under cut which is engaged by the retentive lamellae of the female. If a spacer is used during fabrication, this attachment will be resilient, without the spacer, it will be non-resilient.

Advantages

The Dalla Bona attachment is a relatively trouble free attachment that is simple to use, fabricate and maintain. It will be considered rather than the cylindrical form.

1. Their overall length varies between 3.3 millimeters (cylindrical) to 3.7 millimeters (spherical), so it is suitable for short intra-occlusal spaces.

2. It provides firm, definite retention.

3. It can be processed into the overdenture in the laboratory or mounted in the mouth using auto polymerizing resin.

4. It is less expensive than the Gerber

5. Parallelism of the spherical Bona is less critical than that of the cylindrical Bona.

6. The male posts can be duplicated as resin patterns. These can be mounted on coping patterns and cast as a single unit.

Disadvantages

1. The retentive action of the female is very stiff and difficult to adjust

2. The collar that retains the female housing in the prosthesis is too small. Therefore the female may become loose with normal adjustments and use. Often a bar must be soldered to the top of the female (in which case it must be tempered), or slots must be cut into the collar for additional retention.

3. The males must be parallel, particularly in the cylindrical form.

4. There may be some torquing and tipping of the abutment, particularly if forces are applied to the top of the cylindrical stud and if the coping is not perfectly fitted to the denture base.

THE ROTHERMANN ATTACHMENT

The Rothermann consists of a solid stud (that is soldered to the copings) and a clasp like female (that is mounted in the overdenture). Like many stud attachments, it is available in both resilient and non resilient designs. The resilient form has a taller male and is supplied with special spacers. It applicable where interocclusal space is limited, as the non-resilient design has a vertical dimension of just 1.1 millimeter and the resilient just 1.7 millimeter.

The male features a definite undercut on just one side of the cylinder. A scribe line on the occlusal indicates the position of maximum undercut. The male must be soldered to the coping so that this line (and the undercut below it) is positioned facially. This way, the female"s clasp arms will reach around from lingual to engage the undercut and the bar like retentive lug will fall in the lingual portion of the denture. It will not interfere with the tooth set up and will be locked in thicker resin.

Advantages

1. One of its more important features is its extremely low profile

2. It has adequate retention, which is readily adjusted, similar to the clasps of a clasp partial denture.

3. Parallelism of the males is not critical, but should be made closely parallel for best function.

4. The self-soldering center makes it the easiest to solder of all attachments

5. The male posts do not break

6. The female clip is well retained in the resin

7. The male posts are easily duplicated for resin patterns

Disadvantages

1. Chairside insertion of the female is difficult or even hazardous, therefore the females are best processed in place in the laboratory.

2. sufficient denture bulk must be present lingually to secure the female lug

3. A transfer male is available or relining or rebasing, bust proper orientation of this male in the impression material is difficult and error prone.

4. It is difficult to properly block out the male post and female clasp areas, so acrylic will often lock the two together in processing.

MISCELLANEOUS STUD ATTACHMENTS

Ancrofix attachment

The Ancrofix is similar to the spherical Dalla Bona with a rounded male post providing the undercut for retention. The female is processed within the overdenture. The attachment consists of a male base which is soldered to the coping diaphragm, a removable sleeve knob that provides the undercut, the female has adjustable lamellae that engage the male undercut for retention. A Teflon ring covers the female lamellae similar to the Dalla Bona. This attachment is 3.2 millimeters in height. It can be made resilient by removing the small knob located on top of the male stud and by spacing the copings. The male sleeve can also the interchanged with the solid fixation introfix male attachments.

Introfix and Gmur Attachments

A more rigid attachment is required, particularly as support and retention of removable bridgework or overlay partial dentures, as well as for all tooth suppored overdentures.

The inrofix and Gmur attachments satisfy these requirements

1. **The Introfix** : This attachment has a slotted, cylindrical male post that is engaged by the female for frictional retention. It consists (1) a male base (similar to the Ancrofix base); (2) a slotted, removable stud section that screws into the male base (3) A female that fits over the male. It is available in two different sizes – 4.7 millimeters and 6 millimeters in length. Its use is indicated for retaining and supporting fixed removable bridgework, overlay partial dentures, or an all-tooth supported overdenture. Because the male post is interchangeable with that of the Ancrofix, an all-tooth supported introfix pros-

thesis can be connected to a resilient, stress broken Ancrofix over denture.

2. **The Gmur attachment** also is a rigid fixation stud which is indicated for supporting and retaining fixed removable bridgework or overlay partial dentures. The male is a solid one piece cylindrical rod. The female contains a split sleeve that slides over the male post for adjustable frictional retention

Bona Puffer Stud

This stud attachment has a coil spring inside the female with a vertical translation of approximately 0.8 millimeter. This translation is too large for the limited compressibility of most supporting tissues. To compensate for this vertical movement, the copings should be spaced only 0.5 millimeter, thus limiting its action. This attachment can be used when vertical and rotational movement of the prosthesis is a desirable feature. But due to its large vertical height, more than 5 millimeters, its use is limited by the available vertical space.

BAR ATTACHMENTS

Bar attachments consist of a metal bar that splints two or more abutments, and a companion mechanism processed within the tissue area of the overdenture. This mechanism snaps on the bar to retain the prosthesis. Bar attachments are available commercially in a wide variety of forms or they can easily be "custom" fabricated.

The Bar Unit

This bar has parallel walls providing rigid fixation with frictional retention. It can be used for retention with long, medium or short coping but only when the appliance is to be an all tooth supported appliance (i.e. where no stress broken or rotational action is indicated.) It is never used when a bar joint is indicated (when rotational or vertical action is necessary) however, a bar joint can be used whenever a bar unit is indicated.

The bar joint

The action of this attachment provides rotational or vertical movement. It is a stress broken attachment. It has a rounded or semi rounded contour so the retention clip and prosthesis can rotate slightly during mastication.

The bar joint splints the abutments, retains supports and stabilizes the overdenture. And like the bar unit, it can be used with long, medium or short copings. However, unlike the bar unit, a bar joint minimizes forces on the abutments through its stress broken rotation. Since the typical overdenture abutment is extremely weak, the bar joint is generally preferred to the bar unit.

THE DOLDER BAR

An ideal bar attachment is the Dolder bar. It is well designed for splinting two or more abutments to provide support, stability and retention for the overdenture. This bar attachment is manufactured in two forms – a bar joint and a bar unit. It is also available in two different diameters and lengths.

a. The Pear shaped bar joint is designed to provide vertical and rotational action so it is indicated where a stress bro-ken, resilient attachment is desired. It can also be used as a bar unit for an all tooth supported prosthesis by fabricating the overdenture without planned vertical movement.

b. The bar unit is in the form of an inverted U with parallel walls. It does not permit rotational or vertical movement; therefore it only provides retention and support, but maximizes the matricatory load on the abutments.

Overdenture function

Freedom for vertical movement, provided by the auxillary wire spacer and lead foil covering the copings during fabrication, allows approximately 0.5 to 1.0 mm of space for movement during function. At rest, the overdenture sits passively only on the alveolar tissues. A space is present between the bar – coping assembly and the shell-tissue side of the overdenture. There is maximum retention now since the clip engages the bar undercut.

During mastication, the denture moves vertically. Now it is supported by both the alveolar tissues and the root supported coping-bar substructure. No space is present over the bar and copings. The abutment teeth and soft tissue now absorb maximum denture function.

When the supporting tissue is thin, as in the lower arch, the tissue can be compressed only slightly before the prosthesis should rest on the coping-bar substructure. Approximately 0.5 mm space should be provided in this situation. On the more spongy, fibrous resilient tissues, tissue compression is generally greater. A space of approximately one mm may be required.

Adjusting retention

Retention of the overdenture is easily increased or decreased by adjusting the flanges of the shell to provide desirable retention.

Bending the lingual flange will depress the distal base of the denture. Bending the labial flange tends to keep the anterior segment down. These adjustments can be made easily by inserting a sharp instrument between the retentive blades and the denture base and applying slight pressure to bend the flange. This retention should not be ex-

cessive, otherwise excess stresses will be subjected to the substructure and abutments.

The Dolder Bar Unit

The Dolder Bar unit is an excellent attachment when an all-tooth-supported, non-rotational overdenture is desired. This bar design may be indicated if there are numerous abutments. The bar unit is not rounded like the bar joint, but rather has parallel walls. The friction between these walls and the shell provides the retention. Like the bar joint, the Dolder Unit is available in two sizes. The larger has a vertical bar dimensions of four to five mm. The smaller, a vertical dimension of 3.6 mm.

As because the bar unit has parallel walls, the female shell does not flex much during insertion. This means that the unit leaves less open space than the joint where tissue may proliferate.

The Hader Bar system

The Hader system is an excellent bar attachment. Similar to the customized bar, the Hader system consists of a plastic bar pattern with gingival extension and small plastic clips that are processed into the overdenture. This system has some advantages over others; the plastic bar pattern"s gingival ex-tension can be trimmed to conform to the ridge. In addition, worn clips can be easily replaced at chairside using a special seating tool.

Components of Attachment

Components of the Hader system are

1. Plastic bar pattern (1.8 mm diameter, vertical height 5.7 mm)

2. Plastic clips (5 mm long, 3 mm thick, 4 mm high)

3. Modeling riders used in processing to create a slot for the clips

4. Clip seating tool

Advantages of the Hader system

The Hader bar system has some real advantages over other bar systems.

1. The plastic bar pattern is easily adapted to differences in the surfaces of the gingival ridge and gingival curvature

2. The plastic bar pattern simplifies the laboratory technique by eliminating a soldering step

3. Plastic riders give adequate retention and are easily replaced.

4. Its rotational joint action relieves stresses from the abutment teeth.

The main disadvantage of this system is its plastic rider which cannot be altered for additional retention. However, the adjustable metal riders can be used to eliminate this problem. In addition, there is no provision for developing vertical function with the overdenture.

The Gaerny bar

This retention system has been modified from the channel shoulder pin concept. Retention is provided by precise contact between the virtually parallel surfaces of the inner and outer copings, and the similar contact between the connecting bars and sleeves. Pins are not employed. In order to provide an adequate contact area, a crown length of about 5 mm is usually required.

Gaerny (1969) believed that the interdental spaces should be obliterated by small connecting bars between the fixed inner copings. By doing so, he felt the deposition of plaque would be restricted to the overlying removable section and thus easily displaces when that part of the prosthesis was taken out. This connection at gingival level contributed to the rigidity of the substructure and allowed generous vertical space for the removable unit.

The advantage of using plunger type units, where there was limited frictional surface area. Screws were used as seldom as possible, in view of the problems of plaque control around the screw heads and the small niches around the screws. Screws were used only where it was unavoidable due to the path of insertion of the matrix where the abutments were markedly tilted. Intra coronal attachments were employed on distal tilted abutments.

Current opinion favours neither the encroachment of the interdental space, nor the bulky assembled restoration of limited contour. However, extremely successful long term results have been claimed and demonstrated. The patient"s pla-que control must naturally play an important role in the prognosis as indeed it does for any prosthesis.

THE ANDREWS BRIDGE

An interesting development in bar prosthesis was designed by Andres (1966). Unlike other bar systems, these prefabricated units were made of precision machined stainless steel rather than a gold alloy. Very high tensile and yield strengths were claimed for the material so that the bar could be made thin and also occupy minimal vertical space.

Two types of bars were manufactures : a single bar to use anteriorly and a twin bar for gaps. These bars were available in three lengths of three different curvatures. Each curve was a segment of a circle and the combinations allowed adaptation to most clinical situations. Since the bar formed part of the arc of a circle, it simplified reconstruction should a patient lose or damage the removable section.

One of the advantages is its strength, while the curved construction allowed the use of bars anteriorly where the usual straight section could not be employed. For any given situation, Andrews recommended using the bar with the greatest possible curvature, thereby providing a maximum length and hence more frictional surface and greater wear resistance. It also resulted in a more critical path of insertion that reduced the chance of accidental dislodgement of the prosthesis.

The posterior bar provided greater retention and resistance to all dislodging forces, and smaller versions of both anterior single and posterior twin bars were available where vertical space was restricted. As with all other bar prostheses, careful planning was required with particular attention paid to the assessment of vertical and buccolingual space available, together with an examination of the mucosa to be covered by the bar. The small cross section simplified plaque control and design of the restoration.

Single bars could be used for posterior restorations provided it was unnecessary to reduce the height of the bar. This was useful where buccolingual space was restricted, or when the anterior abutment was well forward in the arch. Adjustment for wear was an unusual feature of the unit, for one adjusted the bar rather than the sleeve.

It was claimed that soldering a bar to a gold restoration did not interfere with its corrosion resistance or mechanical properties, but the soldering process itself seemed more complicated than usual. In fact where posterior restorations were concerned a recessed occlusal rest seat was suggested for the abutment teeth to strengthen this critical junction it was recommended that a mechanical lock be prepared in the bar to rest within the contour of the abutment crown. Apart from the mechanical effects of this lock, it also gave a greater area of contact for the solder. As with any bar retained prosthesis the design of the preparation must allow for adequate bulk of metal close to the gingival margin.

Abutment preparations

All types of bar prostheses require a common path of insertion for the fixed section of the restoration, unless an auxillary system has been incorporated. The retention of an abutment is often severely reduced in an effort to align it with others, and consequently the abutment restoration may subsequently loosen under load applied by the removal of the prosthesis.

Intracoronal attachments may be soldered to bar units connecting them to the tilted abutment. The problem here is vertical space for the intracoronal attachment. Secondly, if the gingival section of the attachment is within the crown contour the occlusal section may be well into the pulp chamber if the tooth is markedly tilted. Connectors that screw the bar to the crown in the mouth overcome the pulpal problems, plaque control difficulties way seen where lack of vertical space exists. A telescopic

crown in which the outer section is soldered to the bar does into solve the vertical space complications as the proximal contour of the inner coping would be an unacceptable plaque trap if it were to correct a tilted abutment. Mechanical solutions to the tilted molar may be considered where clinical crown height exceeds 5 mm.

Dislodging forces applied through the bar to the abutment crowns may cause distortion of the restoration, and for this reason partial coverage retainers cannot normally be recommended. Since the bar is soldered to the crowns, a sufficient bulk of metal is required near the margins. A shoulder or chamber preparation adjacent to the bar is recommended, for this will contribute to the strength of the crown margins which are then prone to damage under load.

Correction of bar distortion

When trying a metal casting in the mouth, one may discover a slight rock. If this rock is slight the assembly will need to be split, though it may not necessitate completely remarking the sleeve : it does illustrate the importance of ensuring that the fixed section of the prosthesis fits perfectly before a sleeve is positioned or waxed-up and cast. The bar is split, using a very fine carborundum disc, and the abutments carefully seated on their respective preparations ensuring that there is now no rock. The two sections of the casting are united with impression plaster and the entire casting then removed in an overall locating impression employing impregum. The dies are now placed in their respective castings and the bar soldered in its correct location.

AUXILLARY ATTACHMENTS

Screws

Screw attachments

A screw attachment generally consists of a metal sleeve waxed into the pattern to become an integral part of the cast primary coping, and a screw which passes through the overlying secondary member – such as a crown or bar – to engage the threaded sleeve. A simple screw system such as the Hruschka, locks two units firmly together. It has a very limited use in overdenture prosthetics. It is more ideally used in fixed removable bridgework.

Schubiger Screw Attachment

An excellent screw attachment often used in overdenture technique is the Schubiger. This attachment is a very versatile screw – type system, used with Gerber and bar combinations.

The Schubiger attachment system consists of a threaded stud base, a sleeve that fits over the threaded stud and an internal threaded screw that screws over the stud base, locking the sleeve into position. Its versatility is due to the fact that its screw base is common to the Gerber screw base; it is therefore completely interchangeable. Thus, a schubiger screw stud and bar attachment assembly overdenture can be modified to a Gerber attachment prosthesis. This attachment is indicated when doweled copings are to be splinted with a bar but the abutments are too divergent for a common path of coping insertion. This situation is easily solved with the Schubiger screw assembly. This attachment is considered when copings splinted with a bar may need to be removed at a later time.

This removable feature is desirable when the prognosis of some of the abutments is questionable. Later, when a weak abutment is lost, the bar can be removed. The prosthesis is then modified to a Gerber overdenture.

PLUNGER TYPE ATTACHMENTS

Auxillary retention can be obtained by plunger type attachments like IC, Iposoclip and pressomatic

These attachments have a plunger that engages a small round depression in a coping wall or in the side of a bar. The IC and ipsoclip systems have spring loaded plungers, the IC being the simpler in construction. The plunger of the Pressomatic unit has a rubber cartridge which maintains the pressure on the plunger.

Ipsoclip and Pressomatic attachments

The Ipsoclip consists of a metal plunger, a coil spring, a housing, and a retaining screw. It is available in two forms-a back-end loading and a front-end loading modification for servicing of this attachment.

The Ipsoclip and Pressomatic is available in regular and high fusing metal for soldering, or for direct casting technique with high fusing metal to receive porcelain.

The Ipsoclip can be used to increase the retention of a secondary metal coping over a primary coping, to improve the retention with a flat bar assembly, or to incorporate such attachments into the overlay portion of a telescopic prosthesis.

When the Ipsoclip is incorporated into the secondary coping casting, the back-loading unit is recommended. If the attachment is to be incorporated into the primary coping – into the bar rider – or inside a resin secondary coping – use the front loading unit.

IC attachment

The action and function of this self contained unit is similar to that of the ipsoclip.

An IC attachment is an excellent attachment for increasing the retention of a telescopic overdenture.

Basic techniques

There are two basic techniques for managing the patient with a Zest anchored overdenture

c. The *indirect approach* involves the prior positioning of the females into endodontically treated teeth. Then transfer males are placed into the females and a master impression is taken of the denture bearing areas and the roots with the females fitted with transfer males. The transfer males are withdrawn with the impression, and females snapped over the posts so that a master cast is produced with substitute females accurately positioned on the cast. The overlay prosthesis is fabricated on the casts in such a way that the males become accurately fabricated in the denture base.

d. The *direct approach* involves the prior fabrication of the overlay prosthesis without males. After the overlay prosthesis is delivered to the dentist, the endodontically treated teeth are fitted with the females. The males are then locked into special recesses within the denture directly in the mouth with self curing resin.

Indirect procedure

Steps in the indirect procedure

   13. Examination, diagnosis and treatment planning

   14. Periodontal therapy and endodontics

   15. Prepare the roots of the desired teeth

   16. Insert females in roots of the tooth

17. Place transfer male into cemented females

18. Take master impression for the overlay prosthesis with the withdrawn transfer males in position

19. Place red substitute females or preferably regular females over the males in the impression

20. Pour the impression to produce cast with transfer females locked in position.

21. Take occlusal registration of the teeth

22. Set up and articulate the teeth

23. Place white males on the cast inside the females

24. Process overlay prosthesis with males in place

Root preparation and seating of females

11. For this treatment all periodontal therapy and extractions should be completed several months the initial operative appointment

12. Use a high speed handpiece with a carbide fissure bur to reduce the teeth to approximately 2-3 mm above the gingival tissues initially

13. If endodontics had not been previously completed, it may be accomplished at this time. Only the apical portion of

the root is filled to allow adequate room for the post of the female.

14. Each root surface is now reduced with a diamond bur in the same plane slightly above the gingiva. This adjustment cut is made at right angles to the path of insertion of the overdenture. When reducing, stop at 0.5 to 1.0 millimeter from the gingiva (at its nearest point). This produces the most favorable crown – root ratio, with little danger of the female being below the gingival crest. Remember, the root surface must be high enough to permit a round periphery. The cut and contoured surface should not be submerged below the gingiva. Other wise, the gingiva will proliferate over the abutments.

15. To prepare a recess into the canal drill a six millimeter pilot hole into the canal with a number two round bur. Drill these pilot holes parallel to each other and to the path of insertion. When making the pilot holes where the females are not to follow the root canal, due to differences in the path of insertion and because of the soft tissue and bone undercuts, care should be exercised so as not

to perforate the root wall. When preparing recesses in multiple rooted teeth, do not perforate the pulpal floor.

16. Next, enlarge the occlusal three to four millimeters of the pilot hole with a fissure or number six round bur to a size slightly smaller than the main body of the female. This eliminates excess drilling with the sizing bur.

17. Prepare the female recess with the special diamond sizing bur. It is best to use a reduction gear contra angle handpiece at a slow speed to avoid excessive movement that might over size the recess, or even break the post portion of the drill. If the opening is inadvertently made too large so the female does not fit snugly, fill the recess with amalgam or a composite filling material and re-prepare. If the canal cannot be followed, remove both the post portion of the drill and the female, or use the mini drill and mini female. The hole should be drilled so that a very, very slight recess is also created on the occlusal root surface with the disc portion of the drill. The female will fit into this recess like an inlay.

18. The female portion is now ready to be cemented into the root. Mix, the crown and bridge cement to the proper consistency for cementing an inlay. Introduce cement deep into the recess with a lentulospiral drill. Next, insert a male attachment into the female with the centering sleeve in position. Add cements to the female, and using the inserted male as a handle, insert the female into the recess. Keep firm pressure on the male until initial set of the cement.

19. After final set of the cement, remove the male post and all excess cement.

20. The root surface is now ready for final preparation and finishing. With a fine diamond bur, remove all sharp corners at the root periphery. Contour, shape and drill toward the gingival margin, but end this contour and root margin approximately 0.5 millimeter above the gingiva. Finally, polish the root surface with appropriate discs and rubber wheels.

Indirect procedure for processing males into the denture

16. After females have been cemented into the roots, the blue transfer posts, with their centering sleeves, are now in-serted into the females in each root. These male posts have slightly less retention than that of the white males, and will be withdrawn easily with the impression.

17. On a previously fabricated study cast, construct a custom tray for a mater impression. Drill holes through the tray over the area of the male posts. These holes minimize possible distortion or dislodgement of the male transfer posts.

18. Since the teeth are reduced to the gingival crest, the arch can be treated as if it were edentulous. Therefore, the tray is muscle trimmed with molding compound to produce an accurate record of the peripheral soft tissue attachments. A master impression may be taken with a zinc oxide impression paste; or even rubber base impression material. Record the denture bearing ridge area and the roots with their females. The transfer posts are then withdrawn within the impression material. This impres-

sion can be made with the impression material of your choice.

19. When the impression is removed, you will notice the ends of the male posts extending out of the impression materi-al. Place spare females or the red substitute females over the ends of these transfer males. These females must be snapped firmly over the posts, but with care so as not to dislodge the males.

20. Pour the cast using the impression, with the transfer females locked securely in place. The transfer females now become an integral part of the master cast.

21. The master cast for the fabrication of the overdenture is now completed.

22. This master cast is used to fabricate an occlusal tray with wax rims for occlusal registration. This occlusal tray may be a shellac tray, a tray made of self curing resin, or even the metal framework used as part of the final prosthesis.

23. For added retention and stability when you take occlusal records, the tray may be fitted with the white Zest males.

To do this, place a hole in the tray over each transfer female to receive the white male posts. Lock the male to the tray or metal framework, with a hard wax or self curing resin. Use of the white males during occlusal registration also aids in the set-up of the denture teeth.

24. Occlusal records are now taken with the technique of your choice.

25. The occlusal records are used to articulate the casts on an appropriate articulator.

26. Before set up of the denture teeth, need is to insert the white male firmly into each female. Push down each centering sleeve to accurately position each male. This makes the ball of the male to firmly engage the female undercut for maximum retention.

27. Bock out all undercuts around the roots with plaster.

28. Set up the denture teeth. The denture set up is then checked in the mouth for occlusion and any esthetic modification.

29. Wax, festoon, flask, pack and finish as you would any conventional complete denture

30. Remove the centering sleeve and excess flash from around each male post. The overdenture is now ready for insertion.

Direct technique

In the direct technique, the overdenture is first fabricated without the Zest males. The females are placed into the abutments, the males snapped into the females, and then locked directly into the overdenture in the mouth. The recess inside the overdenture to receive the males either can be prepared chairside by the dentist, or processes into the overdenture using special male spacers. The following procedure describes the direct technique using male spacers to prepare a recess inside the overdenture to receive the male directly in the mouth.

18. Using the procedure of your choice, take a master impression of the denture bearing ridge areas and existing dentition. The resulting cast will be treated similar to that for an immediate denture insertion.

19. Fabricate custom trays for recording the occlusal registration. Mount the casts on an appropriate articulator.

20. Trim the teeth on the cast to simulate the reduced abutments. Remove the teeth on the cast that are to be extracted later.

21. Using a number forty two drill in a straight handpiece, prepare a hole in the cast of each root that will be fitted with a Zest female. Following the long axis of each tooth, drill the holes parallel to the path of insertion.

22. Insert the special red male spacers into these holes. The spacers assist in the setup of the teeth by providing adequate room for the nylon male. If the holes are drilled correctly, the male spacers should be in correct position over each root. The spacers will be removed after the overdenture is processed, leaving a recess in the tissue side of the denture to accommodate the hub of the white male. You may make adjustments to these recesses, or to the nylon male, if necessary.

23. Set up the denture teeth, articulate, wax, and festoon as you would a conventional complete denture.

24. The denture is half flasked, full-flasked, processed and polished with the spacer in place.

25. Remove the male spacers leaving recesses within the overdenture base to receive the male posts. The overdenture is now delivered to the dentist for insertion.

26. Now the teeth must be prepared to receive the Zest females. The endodontically treated teeth are prepared to receive the females as described earlier. The females are cemented and the denture is ready for insertion and positioning of the male posts.

27. Any teeth to be removed should be extracted at this time.

28. Next, test the fit of the overdenture to be certain that it sits passively on the tissues when it is in position. If any rocking is present, remove any denture material that may be impinging upon the prepared roots or the females.

29. Place a small amount of Vaseline into the females before inserting the males. This prevents self curing resin from getting into the females. Snap the white nylon male, with its centering sleeve, into the cemented female until a definite snap is felt. The centering sleeve must be

firmly seated into the female. This sleeve serves to position the male in proper alignment to engage the female under cut and prevents acrylic resin from entering the female.

30. Insert the denture to be certain it sits passively over the male hub. If it does not, trim the hub or enlarge the male recess inside the overdenture until it does sit passively.

31. Remove the denture. With a small brush paint a small amount of self curing acrylic resin around and particularly under the protruding male hub.

32. Place a small amount of resin into the recess in the tissue side of the overdenture

33. Carefully insert the denture into position. The patient should be instructed to gently close into occlusion and to hold this position until the acrylic resin hardens. Thus, the male is processed in place by the self curing resin with the denture in occlusion.

34. After the acrylic has cured, remove the overdenture, trim excess flash, and remove the centering sleeves. The overdenture is now ready for use.

MINI ZEST ANCHORAGE

The mini zest is smaller than the regular Zest, being approximately 3.25 millimeters in length. Because of this, it is often more applicable in the following situations.

3. It should be used with smaller diameter roots, such as upper laterals, some bicuspids roots, lower anteriors, and in the pulp chamber of multi rooted teeth.

4. It may also be used when the pulpal chamber of teeth is very divergent from the path of insertion.

RELINING AND REABASING PROCEDURS

Torquing will cause severe damage to the remaining supporting abutments. Unstable overdentures must be relined or rebased. If severe undercuts are present in the overdenture, trim the inside of the denture flange sufficiently to remove these undercuts. Remove all male attachments and ream out additional denture base to provide room from impression material and new Zest males. Place blue transfer posts into the females. The males should be accurately positioned with the centering sleeves, as described earlier. Reposition the denture in the mouth to assure that the denture sits passively over the male posts. If not, remove additional acrylic resin over each post, or trim the hub of the males. Remove the denture, dry it thoroughly and then paint an adhesive material inside the overdenture. Take a relining impression with the material of your choice. Have the patient ease gently into occlusion as you border mold the denture by muscle trimming. When the impression material sets, remove the denture. The male posts will be retained within the impression material. Place transfer females over each male. Pour the impression with stone material and trim the hard cast base. Accurately mount the cast with the retained overdenture in a relining jig. Separate the relining jig, leaving the incisal and occlusal teeth imprint in the upper member, and the cast on the lower member. Remove the cast from the jig and pry off the overdenture. Remove the denture teeth and insert them in their respective plaster indexes. Place white Zest males into the transfer females locked in the master model. Position the centering sleeve and block out all root undercuts with plaster. Reposition the cast on the relining jig and close the jig with the teeth in position. Trim the male hub if it hits against any denture teeth. Wax the teeth into position. Wax up the denture base and complete the overdenture as described earlier.

Replacement of broken male posts

Often when the soft or bony tissue undercuts are excessive, it is difficult for the patient to accurately insert the overdenture. Here, insertion will cause excessive flexing of the male and thus encourage breakage. Occasionally the patient will develop a habit of biting the overdenture in place. This is a bad habit since the chances of breaking male posts are increased.

Breakage or premature wear of the male posts, is usually due to causes like poor occlusion, over extended denture flanges misaligned females, an inaccurately fitting overdenture or where the alveolar process has resorbed excessively. Replacing the male posts should not be done without correcting the cause of the excessive wear; otherwise, breakage will continue.

Replacing the males

9. Remove the male post from the denture base. Remove additional acrylic to provide room for the new male post.

10. Insert a male into the female

11. Inset the overdenture to be sure it fits passively over the male.

12. Remove the overdenture and the male post

13. Place a small amount of Vaseline into the female, insert the male firmly into place. Align the male by firmly seating the centering sleeve.

14. Place a small amount of self curing resin around and under the hub of the male post and a minimal amount into the over denture recess.

15. Insert the overdenture and have the patient close lightly into occlusion until the acrylic resin cures

16. Remove the overdenture from the mouth. Remove the centering sleeve and any excess acrylic flash. The overdenture is now ready for insertion.

Stud attachments

Stud anchorage systems are particularly useful as retainers for overlay prostheses. They are versatile in design and application.

Studs are generally used on short copings, where they may be mounted on independent abutments or placed strategically along a span of splinted abutments. A wide variety of studs are available, permitting the dentist to limit and redirect the maximal loading on the mucosa and the abutments.

A stud may be resilient (and thus permit a slight vertical movement) or non resilient. Both resilient and non resilient studs may also offer "hinge freedom" in which the prosthesis rotates much like a bar joint.

Stud attachments may be considered for some of the following conditions

11. For retention, stability and support for an overlay prosthesis.

12. On individual short copings with adequate bone support

13. On individual short copings too distant from each other for use with bars.

14. For strategic placement on a splinted span of short cop-ings

15. For strategic placement on splinted copings when a loss of an abutment is anticipated

16. Where vertical space is limited

17. For use with copings under the denture bases of partial dentures

Use of resilient stud

A resilient attachment permits the tissue to compress slightly before any load is transmitted to the abutment. It is usually preferred.

9. For tissue tooth supported prosthesis

10. When functioning opposite natural dentition

11. When functioning against a non resilient appliance (do not use opposite another resilient appliance).

12. When there are only a few abutments

13. When abutments have minimal bone support

14. To compensate for tissue resorption, ill fitting pros-thesis, or errors in substructure cementation

15. When multi directional (stress broken) action is desirable

16. When there is a minimum denture base

USE NON RESILIENT STUD ATTACHMENT

A non resilient attachment will not allow vertical movement (however, it may permit rotation). It is preferred.

9. With strong abutments having maximum bone support.

10. When functioning against a resilient prosthesis

11. When a large, well fitting denture base is possible

12. When no vertical movement is indicated

13. When an all tooth supported prosthesis is desired

14. When a tooth tissue supported appliance is desired

15. When there is little interocclusal space

16. Opposite a complete denture

Other stud attachments

10. Dalla Bona

11. Introfix

12. Ancrofix

13. Gerber

14. Gmur

15.   rotehrmannn

16.   Huser

17.   Schubiger

18.   Ceka

The Gerber attachments and its functions

The Gerber stud system is a versatile stud attachment used routinely. It consists of a male post soldered to the coping and a retentive female secured within the denture base of the overlay prosthesis. The Gerber attachment is furnished into two different types – a resilient and non resilient form. The male post consist of two parts –a threaded base, which is soldered to the diaphragm of a coping, a removable sleeve with a retentive undercut. The resilient female consists of a female housing copper shim, coil spring, a spring retaining sleeve, C-spring, and threaded retainer. The non resilient female has no copper shim, spring coil or spring retaining sleeve. Convenient tools are also used in the fabrication.

Clinical and Technical procedures

13. Examination, study casts, diagnosis, treatment planning

14. Prophylaxis, soft tissue curettage, home care instructions

15. Fabrication of interim overdenture on study casts

16. Reduction of clinical crowns

17. Initial endodontic therapy (may be completed)

18. Extractions

19. Completion of periodontal therapy

20. Insertion of interim overdentures

21. Final endodontic therapy (if not completed)

22. Operative appointments

23. Laboratory procedures

24. Insertion of prosthesis

Non-resilient Gerber

The non-resilient Gerber attachment technique is similar to that described above but with one exception. As it is non-resilient, the overdenture and female rest on the tissues, copings and male posts in a passive position, no spacing is necessary.

Advantages of the Gerber attachment

6. It provides adequate retention, stability and support

7. All of its post sleeves are interchangeable and replaceable, with the exception of the male screw base.

8. Its retention is light and easily adjustable with springs ad-justable and readily replaced

9. It can be processed directly into the overdenture or positioned in the mouth with auto-polymerizing resin.

10. It can be used in conjunction with bars, especially when used with the Schubiger screw base.

Disadvantages of Gerber attachment

6. It is a complex attachment and maintenance problems are relatively common. The male sleeve may become loose. The internal parts of the female may dislodge when the retaining screw unthreads.

7. Its large vertical dimension makes it impractical for minimal intraocclusal space

8. It requires an assortment of tools for fabrication and maintenance

9. The attachments must be parallel

10. The Gerber permits very little rotational action, so torquing of abutment teeth will occur with alveolar resorption.

DALLA BONA ATTACHMENT

Dalla Bona is a simple stud attachment making an excellent overdenture attachment, available in a resilient or non-resilient series. It is useful when there is minimal vertical space and where rotation, resilience and retention are desired. It consists of a single piece male stud soldered to the coping and a single unit female processed within the denture. It is available in two types : cylindrical and spherical. One form even has an internal coiled spring much like the resilient Gerber. This spring much like the resilient Gerber. This Spring helps control vertical movement.

3. Cylindrical Dalla Bona

The cylindrical male post has parallel walls without an undercut. The female lamella fits snugly over the male posts, providing frictional retention. A PVC ring fits around the female lamellae. This aids in fabrication, and permits the lamellae to flex. The cylindrical Dalla Bona must be parallel, therefore, the male posts must be assembled using a paralleling mandrel and suveyor.

4. Spherical Dalla Bona

The spherical Dalla Bona is similar to the cylindrical, but the male post is spherical. This sphere provides a retentive under cut which is engaged by the retentive lamellae of the female. If a spacer is used during fabrication, this attachment will be resilient, without the spacer, it will be non-resilient.

Advantages

The Dalla Bona attachment is a relatively trouble free attachment that is simple to use, fabricate and maintain. It will be considered rather than the cylindrical form.

7. It provides firm, definite retention.

8. It is less expensive than the Gerber

9. Their overall length varies between 3.3 millimeters (cylindrical) to 3.7 millimeters (spherical), so it is suitable for short intra-occlusal spaces.

10. It can be processed into the overdenture in the laboratory or mounted in the mouth using auto polymerizing resin.

11. Parallelism of the spherical Bona is less critical than that of the cylindrical Bona.

12. The male posts can be duplicated as resin patterns. These can be mounted on coping patterns and cast as a single unit.

Disadvantages

5. The retentive action of the female is very stiff and difficult to adjust

6. The collar that retains the female housing in the prosthesis is too small. Therefore the female may become loose with normal adjustments and use. Often a bar must be soldered to the top of the female (in which case it must be tempered), or slots must be cut into the collar for additional retention.

7. The males must be parallel, particularly in the cylindrical form.

8. There may be some torquing and tipping of the abutment, particularly if forces are applied to the top of the cylindrical stud and if the coping is not perfectly fitted to the denture base.

THE ROTHERMANN ATTACHMENT

The Rothermann consists of a solid stud (and a clasp like female (that is mounted in the overdenture). Like many stud attachments, it is available in both resilient and non resilient designs. The resilient form has a taller male and is supplied with special spacers. It applicable where interocclusal space is limited, as the non-resilient design has a vertical dimension of just 1.1 millimeter and the resilient just 1.7 millimeter.

The male features a definite undercut on just one side of the cylinder. A scribe line on the occlusal indicates the position of maximum undercut. The male must be soldered to the coping so that this line (and the undercut below it) is positioned facially. This way, the female"s clasp arms will reach around from lingual to engage the undercut and the bar like retentive lug will fall in the lingual portion of the denture. It will not interfere with the tooth set up and will be locked in thicker resin.

Advantages

8. One of its more important features is its extremely low profile

9. It has adequate retention, which is readily adjusted, similar to the clasps of a clasp partial denture.

10. Parallelism of the males is not critical, but should be made closely parallel for best function.

11. The self-soldering center makes it the easiest to solder of all attachments

12. The male posts do not break

13. The female clip is well retained in the resin

14. The male posts are easily duplicated for resin patterns

Disadvantages

5. Chairside insertion of the female is difficult or even hazardous, therefore the females are best processed in place in the laboratory.

6. sufficient denture bulk must be present lingually to secure the female lug

7. A transfer male is available or relining or rebasing, bust proper orientation of this male in the impression material is difficult and error prone.

8. It is difficult to properly block out the male post and female clasp areas, so acrylic will often lock the two together in processing.

BAR ATTACHMENTS

Bar attachments consist of a metal bar that splints two or more abutments, and a companion mechanism processed within the tissue area of the overdenture. This mechanism snaps on the bar to retain the prosthesis. Bar attachments are available commercially in a wide variety of forms or they can easily be "custom" fabricated.

The Bar Unit

This bar has parallel walls providing rigid fixation with frictional retention. It can be used for retention with long, medium or short coping but only when the appliance is to be an all tooth supported appliance (i.e. where no stress broken or rotational action is indicated) It is never used when a bar joint is indicated (when rotational or vertical action is necessary) however, a bar joint can be used whenever a bar unit is indicated.

The bar joint

The action of this attachment provides rotational or vertical movement. It is a stress broken attachment. It has a rounded or semi rounded contour so the retention clip and prosthesis can rotate slightly during mastication.

The bar joint splints the abutments, retains supports and stabilizes the overdenture. And like the bar unit, it can be used with long, medium or short copings. However, unlike the bar unit, a bar joint minimizes forces on the abutments through its stress broken rotation. Since the typical overdenture abutment is extremely weak, the bar joint is generally preferred to the bar unit.

THE DOLDER BAR

An ideal bar attachment is the Dolder bar. It is well designed for splinting two or more abutments to provide support, stability and retention for the overdenture. This bar attach-

ment is manufactured in two forms – a bar joint and a bar
unit. It is also available in two different diameters and lengths.

a. The Pear shaped bar joint is designed to provide vertical
and rotational action so it is indicated where a stress
broken, resilient attachment is de-sired. It can also be used as
a bar unit for an all tooth supported prosthesis by fabricating
the over-
denture without planned vertical movement.

b. The bar unit is in the form of an inverted U with parallel walls. It does not permit rotational or vertical
movement; therefore it only provides retention and
support, but maximizes the matricatory load on the
abutments.

Typical Dolder Bar Treatment

1. Endodontics, extractions and periodontal surgery are to
be completed prior to starting the operative process.
Tooth preparations are to be started only after healing

2. With a carbide or diamond fissure bur mounted in a high
speed handpiece, reduce the endodontically treated cus-
pids to one to two millimeters above the gingiva.

3. Now use a diamond bur to prepare the abutments with a bevel or chamfer margin

4. An X indentation was cut into the occlusal surface of each rooth with an inverted cone bur or with the corner of a flat end diamond bur. The strength of the coping diaphragm is increased by the added thickness provided by the indentation. The thinner the coping diaphragm the better the crown root ratio.

5. Retention of the gold casting on the root is an important considerations. Short copings have minimal frictional retention so some auxillary coping retention is imperative. The copings can be retained with posts, parallel or non parallel pins, or a combination of both.

6. Enlarge the canal opening with a number six or eight bur to one half of the bur head depth. This adds strength to the dowel casting union here.

7. Fabricate a customized impression tray on the study casts. Prepare holes in the tray over the root preparations. The impression posts will pass through these holes.

8. Take a muscle trimmed impression of the teeth and soft tissue areas. The previously positioned impression posts are withdrawn with the impression.

9. The impression is poured in stone to produce a master cast with removable dies. Before removing the impression from the casts, carefully remove the impression material over the impression posts.

10. Gently remove the impression posts with a hemostat before removing the master cast from the impression. This will eliminate any danger of fracturing the stone dies.

11. Trim the dies of the master casts, place plastic posts in the dies, shorten the posts and flatten them with a hot spatula. These posts should extend four to five millimeters beyond the dowel canal opening.

12. Lubricate the dies and wax the patterns for short copings

13. Sprue, invest and cast the copings. The copings are finished, but are left with a short section of the sprue on each casting which will be removed later. These retained sprue posts aid in the assembly of the bar to the copings for sldering.

14. Mount the casts on an articular with appropriate intra occlusal records obtained with custom trays and wax occlusal rims

15. Set up the denture teeth and check with the patient for occlusal harmony, vertical dimension and esthetics.

16. Cut the bar to fit between the copings. The bar should be positioned slightly lingual to allow room for the anterior teeth but not too far to interfere with tongue action. If the bar is positioned too far labially, the anteriorly positioned teeth will give the lower lip a very poor esthetic appearance.

Adapt the bar closely to the crest of the alveolar ridge by grinding the gingival portion. The bar should also be positioned horizontally. When the arch is tapering, either bend the bar or cut and solder the bar to conform to the curvature of the arch.

17. To aid in orienting the bar correctly, the previously set up anterior teeth can be indexed with a plaster core.

18. Connect the bar to the copings (the short sprue stubs help here) with Duralay, or sticky wax. Invest and solder

to the copings. Polish the substructure and place on the master cast for assembly.

19. Retention of the overlay prosthesis is provided by the retentive shell processed in the tissue side of the denture base. Cut the shell to fit against the proximal surface of each coping. This retentive shell is fabricated with perforated wings to lock the clip into the denture base).

20. The metal spacer is positioned over the bar and the retentive shell is snapped on the bar securing the spacer. Since this Dolder bar joint is a resilient attachment, when the spacer is removed later, the prosthesis will be spaced for vertical movement.

21. Space must also be provided over the copings. This space over the copings and between the denture base is provided in this manner before the denture teeth are set up, there to four thickness of X-ray foil are adapted over each coping. All spacers will be removed after the overdenture is processed.

22. Block out all undercuts around the copings with plaster and cover the flanges of the retentive shell. If this is not

done properly, acrylic resin processed against the shell will prevent the female retentive areas from flexing. This will eliminate its retentive action. It is of utmost importance that this blocking out process not be excessive. Otherwise, spaces between the denture base and soft tissues will be left where gingival tissue may proliferate.

23. With a small brush, sparingly paint a semi-dry mix of autopolymerizing acrylic resin (such as Duralay) to cover the end of the spacer and shell. This prevent processed denture acrylic being forced into this space locking the bar and shell assembly together. The processed resin will lock the coping bar assembly to the overdenture. The prosthesis may be damaged while removing this resin. Occasionally the coping bar assembly may even be bent.

24. use the stone index to reposition the anterior teeth and complete the denture set-up. Be certain that the blocking out plaster does not interfere with positive seating of the anterior teeth. Trim any of the plaster that may interfere with the positioning of the denture set up.

25. The denture is waxes, festooned, flasked, processed and finished. The coping bar assembly is removed but the retentive shell is retained within the tissue side of the denture. The lead foil, and auxillary spacer, as well as any excess acrylic is carefully removed.

26. Cement the Dolder bar / coping assembly into position. The overlay denture is inserted for use.

Overdenture function

Freedom for vertical movement, provided by the auxillary wire spacer and lead foil covering the copings during fabrication, allows approximately 0.5 to 1.0 mm of space for movement during function. At rest, the overdenture sits passively only on the alveolar tissues. A space is present between the bar – coping assembly and the shell-tissue side of the overdenture. There is maximum retention now since the clip engages the bar undercut.

During mastication, the denture moves vertically. Now it is supported by both the alveolar tissues and the root supported coping-bar substructure. No space is present over the bar and copings. The abutment teeth and soft tissue now absorb maximum denture function.

When the supporting tissue is thin, as in the lower arch, the tissue can be compressed only slightly before the prosthesis should rest on the coping-bar substructure. Approximately 0.5 mm space should be provided in this situation.

Adjusting retention

Retention of the overdenture is easily increased or decreased by adjusting the flanges of the shell to provide desirable retention.

Bending the lingual flange will depress the distal base of the denture. Bending the labial flange tends to keep the anterior segment down. These adjustments can be made easily by inserting a sharp instrument between the retentive blades and the denture base and applying slight pressure to bend the flange. This retention should not be excessive, otherwise excess stresses will be subjected to the substructure and abutments.

The Dolder Bar Unit

The Dolder Bar unit is an excellent attachment when an all-tooth-supported, non-rotational overdenture is desired. This bar design may be indicated if there are numerous abutments. The bar unit is not rounded like the bar joint, but rather has parallel walls. The friction between these walls and the shell provides the retention. Like the bar joint, the Dolder Unit is available in two sizes. The larger has a vertical bar dimensions of four to five mm. The smaller, a vertical dimension of 3.6 mm.

As because the bar unit has parallel walls, the female shell does not flex much during insertion. This means that the unit leaves less open space than the joint where tissue may proliferate.

General technique

The bar unit fabrication technique is virtually the same as that using the bar joint but with these exceptions.

1. No spacer is placed over the bar. The clasping shell fits directly on the bar.
2. No spacing is necessary over the copings.

3. Parallelism of the bar is more critical than with the Dolder joint.

4. A special paralleling mandrel is used to parallel the bar unit.

There are many other bar systems available commercially, such as the Hader bar, Octalink, Ceka, Ackerman, M.P. Channels and C.M. Bars. In addition, bars can be "customized", using a variety of techniques. Commercial retentive clips can be used with these customized bars.

Resin Patterns

Resin patterns of Dolder bar joint or unit make excellent customized patterns. The Dolder joints shell itself can be used as a mold to form a bar. The technique, is fast and inexpensive and particularly applicable where there are irregularities in the alveolar ridge. Simply selected the size shell that corresponds to the bar to be fabricated and lubricate the inside with Masque or silicone spray. If a bar joint pattern is to be produced, bend the flanges together slightly. This will form a "pear shaped" pattern. If a bar unit pattern is desired, spread the flanges so as to produce a parallel-walled resin patterns. Fill the shell with Duralay. After it hardens, remove the Duralay bar and use it as a pattern. If there are irregularities in the ridge, add was to the gingival portion of the resin bar pattern until the bar is in light tissue contact.

Since the shell is used to form the bar, a good male / female fits is virtually assured, and you can wax the directly to the copings for a one-piece casting.

Retentive clips used with customized bars

Numerous metal clips are available to fit customized bars: Ackerman clip, Hader bar metal rider, Baker clip and the Dolder bar shell. These clips can be modified or adjusted to fit the bar, or the bar can be shaped to fit the retentive clip. With a ten or twelve gauge bar made from a round wax pattern, use the metal hader rider, Ackerman or Baker clip. If a clip normally used with a twelve gauge bar is to be used with an eight or ten guage bar is to used with an eight or ten gauge round customized bar, the wax bar pattern should be softened and shaped to a smaller diameter to fit the clip. Such a wax pattern can even be given a "pear-shape" (similar to a Dolder bar joint). The metal riders used with the Hader bar system are designed to allow rotational action without vertical translation. The disadvantage of the metal Hader rider is its ability of provide both rotational and vertical overdenture function.

The Hader Bar system

The Hader system is an excellent bar attachment. Similar to the customized bar, the Hader system consists of a plastic bar pattern with gingival extension and small plastic clips that are processed into the overdenture. This system has some advantages over others; the plastic bar pattern"s gingival ex-tension can be trimmed to conform to the ridge. In addition, worn clips can be easily replaced at chairside using a special seating tool.

Components of Attachment

Components of the Hader system are

5. Plastic bar pattern (1.8 mm diameter, vertical height 5.7 mm)

6. Plastic clips (5 mm long, 3 mm thick, 4 mm high)

7. Modeling riders used in processing to create a slot for the clips

8. Clip seating tool

Hader Bar Technique

1. Take an impression of the prepared abutments, our a cast and trim the dies as you would any bar retained overdenture

2. Wax the coping pattern on the dies.

3. Cut the bar pattern to fit between the coping pattern

4. Heat the bar pattern and adapt it to the ridge curvature

5. Trim the gingival portion of the bar pattern to fit the alveolar ridge

6. Wax the plastic pattern directly to the coping patterns for a single casting, or for greater accuracy, cast separately and solder to the copings.

7. The completed substructure pattern is sprued, invested, cast and finished.

8. Seat the substructure on the cast for completion of the overdenture

9. Position modeling riders on the bar where clips will attach. These riders are removed after the prosthesis is fabricated, leaving a preformed seat to receive the plastic clips for retention.

10. Using plaster, block out all undercuts around copings and below the round portion of the bar.

11. Set up the denture teeth, wax the denture, flask, pack and finish as for any bar overdenture technique.

12. When the overdenture is finished, remove the modeling riders with pliers or a sharp instrument.

13. Use the special seating tool to insert the plastic clip into the slots formed by the modeling rider. The denture is now ready for use.

Relining / Rebasing the Hader Bar system

When relining the hader bay overdenture, remove the plastic riders and several mm of acrylic over all areas of the substructure. This provides sufficient room for the impression material. Reline, or rebase as usual, treating the cast of the bar as discussed above.

Metal clips for retention

Be careful that its retentive flanges are covered with plaster before the prosthesis is processed.

Advantages of the Hader system

The Hader bar system has some real advantages over other bar systems.

5. The plastic bar pattern is easily adapted to differences in the surfaces of the gingival ridge and gingival curvature

6. The plastic bar pattern simplifies the laboratory technique by eliminating a soldering step

7. Plastic riders give adequate retention and are easily replaced.

8. Its rotational joint action relieves stresses from the abutment teeth.

The main disadvantage of this system is its plastic rider which cannot be altered for additional retention. However, the adjustable metal riders can be used to eliminate this problem. In addition, there is no provision for developing vertical function with the overdenture.

The Gaernybar

This retention system has been modified from the channel shoulder pin concept. Retention is provided by precise contact between the virtually parallel surfaces of the inner and outer copings, and the similar contact between the connecting bars and sleeves. Pins are not employed. In order to provide an adequate contact area, a crown length of about 5 mm is usually required.

Gaerny (1969) believed that the interdental spaces should be obliterated by small connecting bars between the fixed inner copings. By doing so, he felt the deposition of plaque would be restricted to the overlying removable section and thus easily displaces when that part of the prosthesis was taken out. This connection at gingival level contributed to the rigidity of the substructure and allowed generous vertical space for the removable unit.

The advantage of using plunger type units, where there was limited frictional surface area. Screws were used as seldom as possible, in view of the problems of plaque control around the screw heads and the small niches around the screws. Screws were used only where it was unavoidable due to the path of insertion of the matrix where the abutments were markedly tilted. Intra coronal attachments were employed on distal tilted abutments.

Current opinion favours neither the encroachment of the interdental space, nor the bulky assembled restoration of limited contour. However, extremely successful long term results have been claimed and demonstrated. The patient"s pla-que control must naturally play an important role in the prognosis as indeed it does for any prosthesis.

THE ANDREWS BRIDGE

An interesting development in bar prosthesis was designed by Andres (1966). Unlike other bar systems, these prefabricated units were made of precision machined stainless steel rather than a gold alloy. Very high tensile and yield strengths were claimed for the material so that the bar could be made thin and also occupy minimal vertical space.

Two types of bars were manufactures : a single bar to use anteriorly and a twin bar for gaps. These bars were available in three lengths of three different curvatures. Each curve was a segment of a circle and the combinations allowed adaptation to most clinical situations. Since the bar formed part of the arc of a circle, it simplified reconstruction should a patient lose or damage the removable section.

One of the advantages is its strength, while the curved construction allowed the use of bars anteriorly where the usual straight section could not be employed. For any given situation, Andrews recommended using the bar with the greatest possible curvature, thereby providing a maximum length and hence more frictional surface and greater wear resistance. It also resulted in a more critical path of insertion that reduced the chance of accidental dislodgement of the prosthesis.

The posterior bar provided greater retention and resistance to all dislodging forces, and smaller versions of both anterior single and posterior twin bars were available where vertical space was restricted. As with all other bar prostheses, careful planning was required with particular attention paid to the assessment of vertical and buccolingual space available, together with an examination of the mucosa to be covered by the bar. The small cross section simplified plaque control and design of the restoration.

Single bars could be used for posterior restorations provided it was unnecessary to reduce the height of the bar. This was useful where buccolingual space was restricted, or when the anterior abutment was well forward in the arch. Adjustment for wear was an unusual feature of the unit, for one adjusted the bar rather than the sleeve.

It was claimed that soldering a bar to a gold restoration did not interfere with its corrosion resistance or mechanical properties, but the soldering process itself seemed more complicated than usual. In fact where posterior restorations were concerned a recessed occlusal rest seat was suggested for the abutment teeth to strengthen this critical junction it was recommended that a mechanical lock be prepared in the bar to rest within the contour of the abutment crown. Apart from the mechanical effects of this lock, it also gave a greater area of contact for the solder. As with any bar retained prosthesis the design of the preparation must allow for adequate bulk of metal close to the gingival margin.

Abutment preparations

All types of bar prostheses require a common path of insertion for the fixed section of the restoration, unless an auxillary system has been incorporated. The retention of an abutment is often severely reduced in an effort to align it with others, and consequently the abutment restoration may subsequently loosen under load applied by the removal of the prosthesis.

Intracoronal attachments may be soldered to bar units connecting them to the tilted abutment. The problem here is vertical space for the intracoronal attachment. Secondly, if the gingival section of the attachment is within the crown contour the occlusal section may be well into the pulp chamber if the tooth is markedly tilted. Connectors that screw the bar to the crown in the mouth overcome the pulpal problems, plaque control difficulties way seen where lack of vertical space exists. A telescopic crown in which the outer section is soldered to the bar

does into solve the vertical space complications as the proximal contour of the inner coping would be an unacceptable plaque trap if it were to correct a tilted abutment. Mechanical solutions to the tilted molar may be considered where clinical crown height exceeds 5 mm.

Dislodging forces applied through the bar to the abutment crowns may cause distortion of the restoration, and for this reason partial coverage retainers cannot normally be recommended. Since the bar is soldered to the crowns, a sufficient bulk of metal is required near the margins. A shoulder or chamber preparation adjacent to the bar is recommended, for this will contribute to the strength of the crown margins which are then prone to damage under load.

Correction of bar distortion

When trying a metal casting in the mouth, one may discover a slight rock. If this rock is slight the assembly will need to be split, though it may not necessitate completely remarking the sleeve : it does illustrate the importance of ensuring that the fixed section of the prosthesis fits perfectly before a sleeve is positioned or waxed-up and cast. The bar is split, using a very fine carborundum disc, and the abutments carefully seated on their respective preparations ensuring that there is now no rock. The two sections of the casting are united with impression plaster and the entire casting then removed in an overall locating impression employing impregum. The dies are now placed in their respective castings and the bar soldered in its correct location.

AUXILLARY ATTACHMENTS

Screws

Screw attachments

A screw attachment generally consists of a metal sleeve waxed into the pattern to become an integral part of the cast primary coping, and a screw which passes through the overlying secondary member – such as a crown or bar – to engage the threaded sleeve. A simple screw system such as the Hruka, locks two units firmly together. It has a very limited use in overdenture prosthetics. It is more ideally used in fixed removable bridgework.

Schubiger Screw Attachment

An excellent screw attachment often used in overdenture technique is the Schubiger. This attachment is a very versatile screw – type system, used with Gerber and bar combinations.

The Schubiger attachment system consists of a threaded stud base, a sleeve that fits over the threaded stud and an internal threaded screw that screws over the stud base, locking the sleeve into position. Its versatility is due to the fact that its screw base is common to the Gerber screw base; it is therefore completely interchangeable. Thus, a schubiger screw stud and bar attachment assembly overdenture can be modified to a Gerber attachment prosthesis. This attachment is indicated when doweled copings are to be splinted with a bar but the abutments are too divergent for a common path of coping insertion. This situation is easily solved with the Schubiger screw assembly. This attachment is considered when copings splinted with a bar may need to be removed at a later time. This removable feature is desirable when the prognosis of some of the abutments is questionable. Later, when a weak abutment is lost, the bar can be removed. The prosthesis is then modified to a Gerber overdenture.

The Schubiger Technique

1. Doweled short copings are fabricated on the trimmed dies.

2. The Schubiger attachment is positioned on each coping (parallel to each other using a paralleling mandrel) similar to that discussed for the Gerber attachment.

3. Each screw base stud is sticky waxed to the coping diaphram.

4. The screw and sleeve are removed. The threaded male base is ready to be invested and soldered to the coping diaphragm. A Gerber soldering cornal is screwed on the screw base to aid soldering.

5. The Schubiger posts are reassembled and the copings are positioned on the cast.

6. A bar is cut to length to fit between the Schubiger sleeves

7. The bar is locked to the sleeves with Duralay or sticky wax, and then removed for soldering

8. The assembled sleeves and bar are invested for soldering. Be careful to see that sufficient investment material is introduced inside the sleeve.

9. The soldered sleeves and the bar unit are screwed over the threaded studs, transforming the single copings to a bar splinted substructure.

10. A bar can be customized with a round sprue wax. Clinically and technically, treatment is similar to any bar prosthesis with clips to produce a bar retained overdenture.

11. The copings are cemented on the abutments individually, and then splinted by screwing the sleeve / bar assembly into place over the threaded studs. This should be done while the cement is still soft. Then it will act as a splinted bar attachments system.

12. If an abutment is lost, the treatment can easily be transformed into a Gerber system simply by unscrewing and removing the bar assembly. The screw bases retained on the copings are then fitted with male Gerber sleeves. Now female Gerbers are locked within the denture base direct-

ly in the mouth or during a rebasing procedure by using Gerber transfer males.

PLUNGER TYPE ATTACHMENTS

Auxillary retention can be obtained by plunger type attachments like IC, Iposoclip and pressomatic

These attachments have a plunger that engages a small round depression in a coping wall or in the side of a bar. The IC and ipsoclip systems have spring loaded plungers, the IC being the simpler in construction. The plunger of the Pressomatic unit has a rubber cartridge which maintains the pressure on the plunger.

Ipsoclip and Pressomatic attachments

The Ipsoclip consists of a metal plunger, a coil spring, a housing, and a retaining screw. It is available in two forms-a back-end loading and a front-end loading modification for servicing of this attachment.

The Ipsoclip and Pressomatic is available in regular and high fusing metal for soldering, or for direct casting technique with high fusing metal to receive porcelain.

The Ipsoclip can be used to increase the retention of a secondary metal coping over a primary coping, to improve the retention with a flat bar assembly, or to incorporate such attachments into the overlay portion of a telescopic prosthesis.

When the Ipsoclip is incorporated into the secondary coping casting, the back-loading unit is recommended. If the attachment is to be incorporated into the primary coping – into the bar rider – or inside a resin secondary coping – use the front loading unit.

When the housing is cast directly into the metal secondary coping, it would be fabricated in this manner.

1. The primary coping is fabricated and positioned on the master cast. This coping must have a flat surface with a round depression which will be engaged by the plunger. If this flat surface on the primary coping is located interproximally, then the front loading unit is used. When lingually, then the back loading unit is used.

2. A pattern is waxed over the primary coping to form a porcelain to metal substructure pattern

3. The housing of the back serviced ipsoclip is waxed into a thick part of the pattern opposite the flat surface of the primary coping.

4. After its internal parts have been removed, the housing is cast with the pattern.

5. The internal parts of the attachment are reassembled after porcelain fabrication.

6. A small round depression must be made in the primary coping to receive the plunger : the flattened surface of the primary coping (which is to receive the plunger) is air brushed with a fine abrasive. This gives this surface a stain like appearance ; the secondary coping is inserted and removed repeatedly. This will "rub" a mark on the primary coping where the small depression is to be drilled. This depression is made at the end of the "rubbed" mark, using a number four bur drill this small depression 0.5 to 1 mm deep.

7. Often it is necessary to make a notch in the primary coping above the hole, or where the plunger strikes first. This helps to guide or force the plunger back into its

housing until it enters and engages the prepared depression. This minimizes wear and possible damage to the plunger.

8. The overlay prosthesis is then fabricated and made ready for use. The plunger is ready to engage the prepared depression to provide added retention for the removable prosthesis.

IC attachment

The action and function of this self contained unit is similar to that of the ipsoclip. It is processed within the denture base of the prosthesis in this manner.

1. Drill a small round depression into the flat proximal surface of a coping (previously fabricated) to receive the plunger.

2. Insert the plunger of the attachment while holding the attachment in a horizontal position and, at right angles to the flat surface, sticky wax the plunger into the depression. This will maintain the unit in position. Cover only the plunger with plaster.

3. Paint tissue colored resin around the sleeve of the attachment and lock the attachment to the frame work. The plaster the covers the plunger will prevent resin from entering the attachment which would render it useless.

4. Now the overlay prosthesis can be fabricated without fear of dislodging the attachment from its position.

5. The fabricated IC attachment telescopic overdenture is now ready for use. The exposed plunger will engage the coping depression when the overdenture is inserted.

An IC attachment is an excellent attachment for increasing the retention of a telescopic overdenture.

REFERENCES

1. D. H. Roberts – Fixed Bridge Prostheses.

2. Ernest L. Miller, Joseph E. Grasso. Removable Partial Prosthodontics.

3. George Graber – Colour Atlas of Dental Medicine Removable Partial Dentures.

4. Glen P. McGivney, Dwight J. Castle Berry. McCracken"s Removable Partial Prosthodontics.

5. Harold W. Preiskel. Precision Attachments in Prosthodontics.

6. John E. Rhoads, Kenneth D. Rudd, Robert M. Morrow Dental Laboratory Procedures Fixed Partial Dentures.

7. John E. Rhoads Kenneth Rudd, Robert Marrow – Dental Laboratory procedures – complete dentures.

8. Kenneth D. Rudd, Robert M. Morrow, Harold F. Eissmann – Dental Laboratory Procedures – Removable Partial Dentures.

9. Sherring Lucas Michael and Martin Paul : Attachments for prosthetic dentistry : Introduction and application.

10. Stewart. Rudd, Kuebbar Clinical Removable Partial Prosthodontics.

11. Tylman"s Theory and Practice of fixed prosthodontics (Seventh Edition).

Periodical literature

1. Ainamo Tukka : precision removable partial dentures with pontic abutment. JPD 1970, 23 : 289-95.

2. Akaltan Funda and Can Gulsen : Retentive characteristics of different dental magnetic systems. JPD 1994, 74(4) : 422-427.

3. Arbree N.S, Galovic G. The use of an attachment system for overlay prosthesis. JPD 1986, 56(1) : 51-55.

4. Becker Curtis M. The Thompson dowel – rest system modified for chrome cobalt RPD frame works. JPD 1978, 39(4) : 384-391.

5. Bengtowall. Precision attachment retained removable partial dentures part I : Technical long term study IJP 1991 ; 4 : 249-257.

6. Benur Z. Semiprecision connector design for distal extension removable partial denture Quint Int. 1988 ; 19 : 879-883.

7. Bercera Geraedo and MacEntee Michael A classification precision attachment JPD 1987;58 : 322-327.

8. Besimo Chrisitian Clinical performance of resin – bonded fixed partial dentures and extra coronal attachments for removable prosthesis. JPD 1997; 78(5) :465-471.

9. Blatterfein Louis The use of the semiprecision rest in RPDs. JPD 1969; 22(3) : 307-332.

10. Bohnenkamp David M. Replacement of a fractured unilateral RPD with a non rigid fixed prosthesis – A clinical report JPD 1996 ; 75(6) : 591-3.

11. Breeding Larry. The effect of stimulated function on the retention of bar – clip retained removable prosthesis. JPD 1996 ; 75(5) : 570-3.

12. Brodbelt Robert HW. A simple paralleling template for precision attachments JPD 1972 ; 27 : 285-288

13. Burns David R. Prospective clinical evaluation of mandibular implant overdentures part II – patient satisfaction and preferences JPD 1995 ; 73 : 364-9.

14. Byrant Ronald A, Faucher Robert R. A locking rod and tube connector. JPD 1983; 49(5) : 647-651

15. Caldarone Charles V. Attachments for partial denture without clasps. JPD 1958; 7(2) : 206-208.

16. Carlyle LW. Magnetically retained implant denture JPD 1986 ;56(5) : 583-586.

17. Charkawi Hussein G. EI and Wakad Mohammed T. EI. Effect of splinting on load distribution of extracoronal attachment with distal extension prosthesis in vitro JPD 1996 ; 76(3) : 315-20.

18. Clayton Joseph A. A stable base precision attachment removable partial denture – Theories and principle DCNA 1980 ; 24 : 1-3.

19. Cohen Brett I. Comparative study of two precision overdenture attachment designs JPD 1976 ; 76 : 145-52.

20. Cohn Louis Alexander The physiologic basis for tooth fixation in precision attached partial dentures JPD 1956; 6 : 22.

21. Cooper Hugh Practice Management related to precision attachment prosthesis. DCNA 1980 ; 24(1) : 45-61.

22. Davis David M, Packer Mark E. Mandibular overdenture stabilized by Astra Tech implants with either Ball attachments or Magnets : 5 years results IJP 1999, 12 : 222-229.

23. Davodi Aria. An implant – supported fixed removable prosthesis with a milled tissue bar and hader clip retention of a restorative option for the edentulous maxilla. JPD 1997 ; 78 (2) : 212-217.

24. Doherty Norine M. In vitro evaluation of resin retained extracoronal precision attachments IJP 1991 ; 4(1) : 63-69.

25. Dolder Eugene J. The bar joint mandibular denture JPD 1961 ; 11(4) : 689-707.

26. Dominici John T. Clinical procedures for stabilizing and connecting O-ring attachments to a mandibular implant overdenture. JPD 1996 ; 76 (3) : 330-3.

27. Dr Burns and Ward JE Review of attachments for RPD design Classification and selection IJP 1990; 3(1) : 90-102.

28. Epstein Daniel, Epstein Philip. Comparison of the retentive properties of six. Prefabricated post overdenture attachment system JPD 1999 ; 82 : 579-84.

29. Federick David R and Caputo Angelo A. Effects of overdenture retention designs and implant orientations on load transfer characteristics JPD 1996 ; 76(6) : 624-32.

30. Gillings Barrie RD. Magnetic retention for complete and partial overdenture part I. JPD 1981 ; 45(5) : 484-491.

31. Gillings Barrie RD. Magnetic retention for overdenture part II. JPD 1983 ; 49(5) : 607-618.

32. Gillings Barrie RD. Samant Asha. Overdentures with Magnetic attachments. DCNA 1990 ; 34(4) : 683-709.

33. Gillis Robert E. Obturator – overdentures retained by nonrigid attachments. JPD 1979 ; 41(2) : 189-192.

34. Gonclaves Aluizio A system of modified attachments for removable partial dentures. JPD 1955; 5(5) : 649-657.

35. Goodkind Richard J. Precision attachment removable partial dentures for the periodontally compromised patient. DCNA 1984 ; 28 : 327-336.

36. Goodman Jerome J and Goodman Herman W. Balance of force in precision free end restorations JPD 1963 ; 13(2) : 302-308.

37. Grosser David. Dynamics of internal precision attachment JPD 1953 ; 3 : 383-401.

38. Guindea Abraham E. A retentive device for removable dentures JPD 1972 ; 27 : 501-508.

39. Handlers martin, Lenchner Nathaniel A retaining device for partial dentures. JPD 1957 ; 7(4) : 483-488.

40. Harris Fred W. Precision dowel rest attachment JPD 1955 ; 5 : 43-47.

41. Herrero Dale. B. Repairing and strengthening a fractured Hadar bar. JPD 1977 ; 77(1) : 90-92.

42. Highton R, Caputo AA. Retentive characteristics of different magnetic systems for dental applications JPD 1986 ; 56(1) : 104-106.

43. Hutcherson J Bernard Practical partial dentures restoration JPD 1955 ; 5(2) : 206-207.

44. Jackson Thomas R and Healey Kent W. Rare earth magnetic attachments in the state of art in removable prosthodontics Quint Int nl 1987 ; 18 : 41-57.

45. Jaggers Joe H. A method of verifying parallelism of preparations for zest anchor attachments JPD 1978 ; 39(2) : 230-231.

46. James Allison G. A self locking posterior attachment for removable tooth supported partial denture. JPD 1955 ; 5(2) : 200-205.

47. James White. Visualization of stressed strain related to removable partial denture abutments JPD 1978 ; 40(2) : 143-157.

48. Joseph Clayton A. A stable base precision attachment removable partial denture Theories and principles DCNA 1980 ; 24(1) : 3-29.

49. Knowles Leroy E. A dowel attachment removable partial denture JPD 1963 ; 13(4) : 679-687.

50. Koper Alex. An intraoral semi precision retainer for removable partial dentures – The Thompson Dowel JPD 1973 ; 30 : 759-68.

51. Kotowicz WE Clinical procedures in precision attachment removable partial denture construction DCNA 1980 ; 24 : 143-166.

52. Lee Kyuho. Double impression procedure for removable partial denture retained with semiprecision attachments – A clinical report JPD 1996 ; 75(6) : 583-7.

53. Lee Ming- Way. O-raing coping attachments for removable partial dentures JPD 1995 ; 74 (3) : 235-41.

54. Leff Alexander Precision attachment dentures JPD 1952 ; 2 (1) : 84-91.

55. Lemon James C. Technique for magnetic placement and orientation of a facial prosthesis JPD 1996 ; 75 :50-52.

56. Lemon James C. Technique for magnetic replacement and silicone facial prosthesis JPD 1995 ; 73(2) :166-168.

57. Leung T, Preiskel. Retention profiles of study type precision attachments IJP 1991 ; 4(2) : 175-179.

58. Levitch Herman C. Physiologic stress equalizer JPD 1953 ; 3(2) : 232-238.

59. Lorenchi Stanley F. Planning precision attachment restorations JPD 1969; 21(5) : 506-508.

60. Markley MR. Broken stress principle and design in fixed bridge prosthesis. JPD 1951 ; 1(4) : 416-213.

61. Marquardt George Dolder bar joint mandibular overdenture – A technique for non parallel abutment teeth. JPD 1976 ; 36(1) : 101-111.

62. McLeod Neil S. A theoretical analysis of the mechanics of Thompson dowel semiprecision intracoronal retainer. JPD 1977 ; 37(1) : 19-27.

63. Mensor Merrill C. Attachment fixation for overdenture part I JPD 1977; 37 : 366-373.

64. Mensor Merrill C. Attachment fixation for overdenture part II JPD 1978; 39 : 16-20.

65. Mensor Merrill C. Clasification and selection of attachemtns JPD 1973 ; 29 : 494-497

66. Mensor Merrill C. the rationale of resilient hinge action stress breakers JPD1968 ; 20(3) : 204-215.

67. Mensor Merrill C. Removable Partial Over Dentures with Mechanical (Precision) Attachments, DCNA 1990 ; 34 (4) : 669-681.

68. Moghadam BK. Scandrett Forest R. Magnetic retention for overdenture JPD 1979 ; 41(1) : 26-29.

69. Naert I. Rigidly splinted implants in the resorbed maxilla to retain a hinging overdenture – A series of clinical reports for upto 4 years. JPD 1998 ; 79(2) : 156-64.

70. O"Connor Randolph P. Use of the split pontic nonrigid connector with the tilled molar abutment. JPD 1986 ; 56(2) : 249-257.

71. Panno Francis V. Crown preparations for semiprecision attachment removable partial denture DCNA. 1985 ; 29(1) : 117-132.

72. Plotnick Irwin J. Internal attachment for fixed treatment removable partial denture. JPD 1958; 8 : 85-93.

73. Riley MA, Williams AJ. Investigations into the failure of dental magnets. IJP. 1999 ; 12 : 249-254.

74. Robinson JE. Magnets for the retention of a sectional intraoral prosthesis. JPD 1963 ; 13(6) : 1167-1171.

75. Rubenstein Jeffrey E. Attachments used for implant supported facial prosthesis – A survey of United States, Canadian and Swedish centers JPD 1995 ; 73 : 262-6.

76. Rudd Kenneth D. An esthetic and hygienic approach to the use of intra coronal attachments as interlocks in fixed prosthodontics . JPD 1998 ; 79(3) : 347-349.

77. Rybeck S Arthur. Simplicity in a distal extension partial denture. JPD 1954 ; 4(1) : 87-92.

78. Saygili Gulbia. Investigation of the effect of magnetic retention system used in prosthesis on buccal mucosal blood flow. IJP 1992 ; 5(4) : 327-332.

79. Schuyler CH. An analysis of the use and relative value of the precision attachments and clasp in partial denture planning. JPD 1953 ; 3 : 711-717.

80. Schuyler Clyde H. An analysis of the use and relative value of the precision attachment of the clasp in partial denture planning. JPD 1953 ; 3(5) : 711-714.

81. Scott William R. A removable telescopic external attachment with an axial rotational joint. JPD 1968 ; 20(3) : 216-225.

82. Scott William R. Laboratory procedures for fabricating the removable telescopic attachment and joint. JPD 1968; 20(3) : 226-234.

83. Setz Juergen. Retention of prefabricated attachments for implant stabilized overdentures in the edentulous mandible. A in vitro study JPD 1998 ; 80(3) : 323-9.

84. Shillinburg Herbet T, Fisher Donald W. Non rigid connec-tors for fixed partial dentures. JADA 1973 ; 87 : 1195-1199.

85. Shohet Harmon. Relative magnitude of stress on abutment teeth with different retainers JPD 1969 ; 21 : 267-282.

86. Stewart BL, Edwards RO. Retention and wear of precision type attachments. JPD 1983 ; 49(1) : 28-34.

87. Tarlow Jeffrey and Rissin Louis. The microring semi-precision attachment for mandibular staple bone implant prosthesis JPD 1982 ; 48(6) : 695-697.

88. Terrell, Wilfrid Hall. Specialized frictional attachments and their role in partial denture construction. JPD 1951 ; 1(3) : 337-350.

89. Thayer HH, Caputo. Occlusal force transmission by over-denture attachments. JPD 1979 ; 41(3) : 266-271.

90. Thayer HH, Caputo AA. Occlusal force transmission by overdenture attachments. Additional studies. IADR Prosthodontic Abstract JPD 1978 ; 39 : 1-55.

91. Thomas Keith F. Free standing magnetic retention for extra oral prosthesis with osseointegrated implants JPD 1995 ; 73(2) : 162-5.

92. Walton Joanne and Ruse Dorin. In vitro changes in clips and bars used to retain implant overdenture JPD 1995 ; 74 (5) : 482-6.

93. Waltz Mark E. Ceka intracoronal attachments JPD 1993 ; 29 : 167-171.

94. Watkinon Adrian C. The replacement of attachment retained prosthesis. Quint Intt. 1987 ; 18 : 759-61.

95. Weintraub Gerald S. Hybrid prosthetic appliances DCNA 1987 ; 31 (3) : 441-456.

96. Williams Arthur G. Technique for provisional splint with attachment JPD 1969 ; 21(5) : 555-559.

97. Williamson Russell T. Retentive bar overdenture clip replacement JPD 1995 ; 74 : 117-8.

98. Winkler Sheldon. A review of extracoronal and intracoronal retainer systems. DCNA 1985 ; 29(1) : 57-66

99. Wolfe Robert E. Extracoronal attachments DCNA 1985 ; 29(1) : 185-198.

100.   Zahler Joel M. Intracoronal precision attachments. 1980 ; 24 (1) : 131-141.

101.   Zinner Ira D. Locking types of semiprecision attachments. DCNA 1985 ; 29(1) : 81-96.

102.   Zinner Ira D. Nonlocking type of semiprecision attachments DCNA 1985; 29(1) : 97.

103.   Zinner Ira D. Precision attachments DCNA 1987; 31(3) : 395-416.

CONTENTS

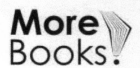
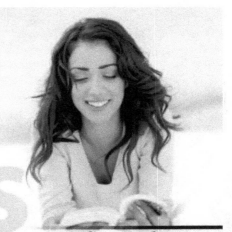
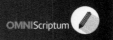

Printed in the USA
CPSIA information can be obtained
at www.ICGtesting.com
LVHW092153260923
759451LV00006B/68

9 786200 529008